CW00822211

The Covid Con;

A Wake

By

courtenay-adam-lawrence

ISBN Number: 9781527273214

Paperback edition (2020)

Once again, I need to dedicate
this book to judy:

the true definition of unconditional love.

You lift my spirit.

Forever, all my love...

Table of contents

The Con.

No Virus;

No Test;

No Contagion.

2020 has proven to be a head-in-a-washing machine year. We've been rinsed (and now being repeated) on full spin.

Suddenly - as planned - it's time for a brave new world, Mr Huxley. A new sell-a-vision, a new 2030 tell-a-vision. All while... Harry fries fish and chips by day, and batters his wife by night. During lockdown.

Being upfront, straight and truthful:

This book will take you from Mary Poppins to Pol Pot e. mouthed.

It will help you live on your feet, not cower on your knees, as the year of fear is now among us.

If you won't take individual responsibility and seek a just remedy... this book won't help.

The way 2020 has been unfolding has taken many by surprise. It has been, and continues to be, disconcerting. There has been an attack on our senses, sensibilities and our humanity.

The sheer volume of news, information and disinformation is bewildering. On any given day if you've fed on the mainstream news you might not know whether you are coming or going. A steady diet of fear can do that to you.

The media is not a reflection of reality. The media is the virus.

As you read this book know that you are in control. I am not forcing you to read it. Do it at your own pace and if it gets too much for you, for any reason, just put it down... and breathe.

You can often forget the same applies when you're reading or watching any of the mainstream (or otherwise) media.

You are the one in control.

"Our deepest fear is not that we are inadequate. Our deepest fear is that we are powerful beyond measure. It is our light, not our darkness that most frightens us." Marianne Williamson.

You don't have to be glued to your television, computer, tablet or smartphone.

Consume what you want and leave alone what you don't want.

You might find this book is a bit frack to bunt and that, in some places, the spalling is appelling. It is a random walk, nothing more; it's the only way the threads could make even a bit of sense. As a full-blown 'covid denier' as one lady labelled me while I was handing out 'covid aware' leaflets.

It is, however, such a serious subject that I state no rights reserved up front to get my word out uncensored. I mean it, due to the criminality and eugenicist tendencies that drive those people hiding behind the actual covid-con-curtain.

It's about people. Seen (and unseen).

The journey to this book started five years ago, when I was phoned by a medical consultant about unnecessary deaths at Noble's hospital on the Isle of Man, where I live happily - when not interfered with. It seems I was the last listening gobshite standing. If the language offends, then covid-19-84 crimes might do more so - I'm hoping - as you read on.

It is some 9 months on now from the locking down of my first book, From Health Heretic To Common Law Advocate, later released on an unsuspecting public on 1st April 2020. I avoided mentioning the Noble's hospital deaths - as it seemed unsporting to do so. But now, with more medical murder on our island, at Abbotswood nursing home, it is finally time to speak up and, more importantly, to man up. Or womb-man up, if you are of an altogether different, but equally concerned, stripe.

If men are from mars and women are from venus, then anything that joins us together, while reducing our angst - must be welcomed. But that is not the division agenda that is running 24/7, while we sleep.

Many of you will have bought and read that book. If you did then, I think, you will already be 'ahead of the game', and certainly ahead of the majority of people; you will have some idea of what goes on behind the scenes and, often, right in front of our faces.

For those who blindly refused to stop and question what I was talking about, I hazard a guess that now some of you must be.

If we were to take a proper gander at some of the unimaginable things that have gone on since, I think you would agree that there is something drastically amiss in our world.

Many people in life, not just authors, prefer to write their own script. To plot their own route. Unfortunately, a few others would prefer to write the script for you to slavishly follow, unquestioningly and obediently. I think it is fair to say they have done their own plotting.

Choice is such a quaint word.

That word 'choice' has become draconianly challenged in 2020. Suddenly George Orwell and covid-19-84 has a ring to it as does, perhaps, even covid-5G. More so, as the EU have said we must only allow peeps to arrange those letters and numbers in selective contexts. The mainstream media and would-be survivors of the world's worst 'pandemic' ever:

lockdown-savvy Sweden's 99.98% survivor-ship;

the UK's catastrophic 99.97% survivor-ship;

and Belgium, being fully investigated by Hercule Poirot, comes in at a genocidally low 99.94% survivor-ship!

The BBC, in their carelessness, gave us fair warning.

A reminder for you that on 9/11 (19 years ago) Jane Standley, repeating a script live on air in New York, reported that the Solomon Brothers' building (WTC-Building 7) had collapsed; luckily predicting its actual bringing down some 23 minutes later. In the 'twin' tower complex. Subsequently, the BBC made no reference to this error and, in fact, pulled their footage from any and all media. And discussion. (refer page 33 From Health Heretic To Common Law Advocate.)

Cover-of-covid is just the new 9/11.

The latter had an enemy without a postcode but with a dark skin.

The former is an enemy everywhere, in anyone, of all skin colours.

In short, a much bigger budget.

Mr Hitchcock.

Two weeks after the US election in 2020, in reference to the film Clash Of The Titans, top licensed legaler Sidney Powell vows to Unleash The Kraken. She authored, Licence to Lie.

Why she, you may ask? Well, she's on team Trump, which has

thousands of testimonies, autographed under penalty of perjury, of voter fraud - in 12 states.

My favourite has to be the ballot cast in the system by the 118 year old, who had actually died in 1984. George.

The postal ballots in their millions allow for mass fraud as even blunt knife Jimmy Carter highlighted years ago. It seems the prime fiddlers are in Pennsylvania and Michigan. The states that didn't allow independent monitoring are clear favourites for the fiddlers stakes... in the 3:22pm at Wincanton, over soft ground. With the jockey (and owner) carrying a bit of weight. The prize is now more than two guineas.

Any Twatter 'fact checkers' reading this will be pencilling in at this point a warning, 'This claim about election fraud is disputed'.

But may we ask Sid, why she no lookie a bit deeper into things? Especially as she followed Rudy on the recent mic' night extravaganza. Rudy, being Mr Giuliani, who was mayor of New York on 9/11/ in 2001.

Fast forward to 2020 and on 9/11 this year he was on CNN, who are not normally viewed as a favourite reporter of all things whole and dandy. But the CNN soft-soaping suited his agenda that day. Just why no one was running over to grab a copy of my report on the original 9/11, I don't know.

Rudy, baby, 9/11 was an inside job and you lot know it.

On 4th July 2019, I'd not only sent my 13 years of research notes to the common law court, but also stateside to Robert David Steele who has, of late, been making some pretty serious accusations of US fraud (of $-trillions), by Wall Street on the minions on main street.

Robert, when he got my document, said it contained information he had never seen. Rumour has it, that he had trained 8,300 C.I.A. operatives and so my already pumped and primed smug-o-meter, went clean through the roof. Although, soon it must be said, my firework fell to earth when I informed him that the black robes he wore in the ITNJ courts had a deeper symbolic meaning than the educational one he'd imagined. All contact severed, m'lud.

Many Looney Tunes™ are being played, and they are not all as good as The Pogues' Fairytale of New York.

Come in number 77 your time is up.

The British army used to engage in armed combat when Hitler was up and at us, and all we had was Captain Mainwaring and two pitchforks. But now the British army has its very own 'troops', pitching in with forked tongues.

There are said to be 4,000 of these people online, fighting the good digital war: of 'domestic terrorists' who question the b/s of the covid-con. More so, as World War III, under the cover-of-covid-context has kicked off.

Can't we just 'control-alt-delete' them and start again with honour? They blindly follow their orders and continue the work of Joseph Goebbels, where he taught:

'If you repeat a lie often enough, people will believe it, and you will even come to believe it yourself'.

Goebbels was certainly the consummate master of propaganda:

'There was no point in seeking to convert the intellectuals. For intellectuals would never be converted and would anyway always yield to the stronger, and this will always be 'the man in the street.' Arguments must therefore be crude, clear and forcible, and appeal to emotions and instincts, not the intellect. Truth was unimportant and entirely subordinate to tactics and psychology'.

Clearly we are witnessing firsthand that truth is unimportant with each passing day.

That, after two months of media terror, a beaten dog licks and likes his captors. Now, as we're almost ten months in to this covid-con it's not just in Stockholm but Stuttgart and Sunderland too.

As it happens, in late October 2020 I travelled off island not to Stuttgart or Sunderland but to Stockholm.

In Manchester, on the outbound leg, I'd met with two friends for dinner; a rather quaint old-fashioned concept I grant you. Food and some life sustaining chat were on the menu. Later, we returned to the car where it now sported a not so natty parking ticket - a yellow and black warning bag attached to the bug screen. Well they, those council lurkers and shirkers, can bugger off, I thought. The energy vampires were soon to receive a bespoke version of the 14 page David Ward v Warrington Borough Council epistle, for their parking piracy scam.

In travelling light, with just one old bag, I'd figured I could get off any plane faster. In travelling as a light being, I also hoped to absorb the vibes and uplifting light of others. But first, it was flight time…

At Manchester airport, the gate lady said I needed a letter (from teacher?). Apparently my Face Covering Exempt badge stating, 'My hidden disability makes me exempt from wearing a face covering' was not enough. Reading ignore-ance and a lack of facts were now fully trending, via the twatterati.

Soon after getting on board for the first flight leg of my journey, a crewman asked me to mask up, as he nose best. I said I was medically exempt and I wouldn't mask scientific truth for him or anyone. Then walkie-talkie Tina rocked up, checking my seat number. Maybe the plane layout was a moveable feast and she was lost. Next up, at the pointy end, I saw a bloke put his suit jacket on with spaghetti on the shoulders - so he must be very important.

In anticipation of what was to follow, I asked the chatty lady in front if she'd mind videoing it, if the Feds arrived looking for plane profit. Spag Bol man duly arrived, and across the aisle a fellow called James, being ever so quick, caught the slight drama in 90 seconds worth of video.

Finally, jacket man cleared off; him being convinced I'm compliant and cleanish, and that I'm happily off to a masked ball - of his choice not mine. Fcukin nazis, ignoramuses and cretins - I was tempted to say, but seeing as we we're both polite I wished him, "peace and love". On camera.

Later, KLM's very owned, Georgia Orwell-De-Klerk, announced, "you are not allowed to film crew or passengers as it violates their privacy" which proved hard to hear as she spoke through her white slave mask. Still, at least a few gilding-ze-lilly numbers would in Georgia's bank account at the endingz of zee month.

The thought nazis weren't done yet...

I was about to get legged over on the second leg, going from Amsterdam to Stockholm. At the gate, I presented my boarding card to the desk scanner. Jumping jack and in a flash it read, in red, 'unable to board'. The David Walliams' 'computer says no' sketch hit my brain. I stood motionless while the lady fiddled with her laptop before handing me back my pass-port and boarding card. Phew, close shave I mused; though unamused.

But there was more…

As I got to the plane, I was stopped at the door by a pursed lip man, "We are aware of your views but do not accept them. They phoned us through. The mask must cover your nose and mouth or we will not let you board". I felt a gentle question coming on and asked, "Can I email you about the issues, individually?". Of course he replied, "No". A quick sending of my one pager, 'No Virus; No Test; No Contagion.' might have helped him. He could start a fire with it, at least, if only his brain wasn't such a damp match.

My first impressions of SwedeLand had me spotting some SS (Stockholm Syndrome) traits, where hope is unwittingly and steadily being extinguished while most snuggle under a max tog duvet. Sweden is prime land for the unfolding agenda, despite (so far) not going lockdown crazy.

There, a slow creep is underway. Granted, few see the coming home prison cell, topped off with clean sheets once a week and three square meals a month. The sustainable comestibles doled out on a square wooden platter. That's where the term 'square meal' comes from - for fans of Shakespeare.

Doled out, too, is a dole handout for the unworked; as jobs are being banned, under the cover-of-covid. As we slip and slide our way into a universal basic income received from the state. For acquiescence.

Once cut free in Stockholm, an evening dinner with Dolores raised my spirit. Group hugs, no masks, no temperature control - whatever were the fellow diners thinking? Next up we were speaking freely to each other and finding common ground across the gathering clans. I even met a fully awakened Irish barrister.

Wonderful, too, to meet the first of the Spanish doctors to

speak out on 'covid' criminality. In previous months she'd been sustained by the videos of Dolores. Later that evening, she cried as they hugged on the walk back to our hotel. At that moment, I was beyond moved to realise what was at stake. I felt my long departed dad on my shoulder.

Next morning, at the hotel, Ole Dammegard was kipping on the sofa - wearing the only pair of shoes he possessed. Quite, clothes and stuff do possess us. I'd followed him for a while, though the Daily Mail, of course, hadn't. His website shines light on the darkness called, as it is, LightOnConspiracies. That Ole had an escape rope outside the back of his Spanish flat, three floors up... shows that when your work is to pre-announce (planned) terrorist acts, your life is fully on the line.

You need a head for heights, and a stomach for the depths of depravity too. Or what bankers, politicians, and stars of staged and screened events get up to. Ole had dug deep on the murder of Olof Palme, the former Swedish prime minister, and found that the smoking guns and building owners had some friends in very high palaces.

At breakfast time I was diving into a yokey egg and coffee, when I met a fellow diner. He introduced himself, "Hello, I'm Niels". Whoa, there, hold the front pages. Although, while holding 'his' research views, he was never permitted even onto the back ones.

It was none other than Dr Niels Harrit, who exposed the residual nano-thermite which helped cut through the 9/11 'twin towers' (as 1000f colder plane gasoline just couldn't be guaranteed to do the job so well). A war on terror needs certainty, damn it! Not big-hat-no-cattle cowboys. No, actually George, it does - it needs Texans. Anyway, over double oeufs and French bread... I got to know another truth-teller and thoroughly good egg - old bean.

Niels and Ole are the ultimate, 'Say your truths, whatever the cost'. Real men with brave hearts.

As, like the virus which is only an issue at certain times, we were now on European time a leisurely breakfast beckoned.

Next up a chat and gentle tones, and smiling face, with Mr Mohammad Adil, him being a Consultant Surgeon. Or former surgeon that should be, since he spoke out on the covid-con way back in April. Despite a thirty year unblemished record, that is, without leaving medical equipment (or welding gauntlets) in the guts of his patients. Being somewhat insightful, he'd noticed that under the skin we are all the same: organs, vessels and tubes. But in the case of the covid-con perpetrators - likely missing a heart.

Later we went to the 'covid-19-84' event in central Stockholm.

When (actual) vaccine researcher Senta Depuydt got on the mic' it was to announce the launch of Children's Health Defense Europe and her work with Robert F Kennedy Jr. Later, over dinner, I learnt that the reason they now inject dogs in their tail is so they can chop off the bit that subsequently gets a tumour.

TV vet Noel Fitzpatrick might fancy speaking up; although, if he does, will likely see a falling workload. We can but hope.

Soon taking to the stage was Dr Ingemar Ljungqvist, who wrote (in Swedish) The AIDS Tabu, an injected 'disease' which he mentioned was fledged in room 451, Fort Detrick, a gain of function, specialist lab - for knocking stuff up. He wasn't done yet with more gain of function info when, coincidentally, it was the recent villains in Wuhan who turned on their 5G masts just over 12 months ago (31st October 2019).

5G is a weapons grade technology which is totally uninsurable;

but necessary? Vital, so adrenochrome junkies can watch and be turned on by their 'films'. Even more coincidentally, Wuhan's 5G was turned on, at Halloween, aligning as it did with mandatory flu vaccine season. No wonder the body does a seasonal detox - and the EU wants a 5G and flu whitewash.

Ingemar was soon doling out more word wizardry, as Tedros Ghebreyesus, the director-general of the WHO dropped the un-cool and un-hip coronavirus moniker, as Teddy knocked one out the park renaming it 'covid', a new and hip name.

Being simple in any language, a name aimed at sheep; or should it be c-ovid, with latin derived ovid, being members of the sheep(le) family? Teddy baby has nothing if not a bit of humour. But as a former terrorist, he's clearly into black humour.

On Saturday night Dr Judy Mikovits was dialled up, dropping in over the pudding... reminding us that Ebola bodies were cremated to stop autopsy evidence. So, actual autopsy cancellations have prior form mirroring the current 'covid' scamdemic cloak - mass graving bodies with a Ferguson tractor.

Judy Mikovits was, for 22 years, based at Fort Detrick US Army Medical Command in Frederick, Maryland. It was all Mary's land, back then. My question to her was simple, "Did the new method of manufacture of major flu vaccines (fluzone, fluad, flucelvax and flumist) in dogs, result in more contamination in particles that some might call coronaviruses?". "Yes, it did", was the answer.

So let's look there first, as the 'covid' pump primer. With 96% of Manx 'covid' deaths being flu vaccinated, an open jury awaits.

It's now early November 2020 and the army has deployed

2,000 troops onto the streets of Liverpool, England. To test you, without any possibility of refusal. If you test positive you get to stay in your own home prison, receive £500 free money and entry onto the National Sick Service track and trace scheme; listed as a disgusting contaminated puss filled enemy of the state folks, aka the likes of Ant and Dec, and Phillip Schofield. What a state.

In the colonies, too, the BMJ has just served one up from down under, and very below the belt it is nowadays in Australia. Those formally rugged and outdoor types are proposing a five year jail term for refusal to have the coronavirus vaccine or face a… $66,600 fine. The devil is not so much in the detail as in the fine.

They're taking the pee, numerically, matron - in plain sight. The lever pullers know all that, the message and messenger crafters - with their three phrase chanty sayings:

1) stay safe 2) stay home 3) snitch on yer 92 year old grannie.

One Messenger they really didn't like, up close and personal, was Melinda. Who spilled the HPV vaccine carnage message all over daytime TV studios. The editor had to hastily get out several mops and buckets, and call in someone - just anyone - to doctor the facts. But well done oh fearless one.

Truth is a messenger that no one can shoot. Given the time, it gets out.

Andy Burnham, was not actually a media darling when, in April 2017 he raised a bloody scandal, in his last speech to the Westminster parliament.

He spoke about the 40 year 'establishment' coverup of NHS contaminated blood. That factor 8 'blood products' were obtained under payment to US 'skid row' providers. It was known then, and it is known now, that they were toxic - so they stopped screening and tragic Magic Johnson like, 'the problem went away'.

But the media was silent.

It should stain the conscience of any society. As it will, when it comes to court, for the current Westminster cronies who are trying to enforce: lock-up, lock-in, lock-step and lockdown by the lock nut nazi's in black, in Manchester. Where Mr Burnham is, for now, a media darling and Greater Manchester mayor.

But, some say, he was acting for the camera while asking for more money to lockdown his people. Andy was holding firm, insisting on 65 million large ones to keep the pubs and clubs swinging.

By 18th October 2020 Andy was landing some good old Oxfordian punches saying the prime minister, Boris Johnson, had engaged in exaggeration of the severity of 'covid-19-84'. Nice, and so in the money - but not for Mancunians.

Besides any exaggerating, in mid October, BoJo was also peddling a lecturnian message of Hands, Face, Space, but no knees and no boomps-a-daisie; they must have bought an early Christmas cracker.

Andy is one of Liverpool's finest, for now on loan to Manchester.

More locally, accounting for the need to keep the lockdown wheels fully greased is Sir Kenny Dalglish. Or 'King' Kenny, as he has been crowned in all his glory - particularly after his majestic compassion following the Hillsborough tragedy. When police falsified 160 witness statements and shamed the whole force. And all of Britain.

The two minute video from VST Enterprises featuring Sir Kenny is worth transcribing:

As everyone is playing in different roles (and shirts) KD = Kenny Dalglish, L-JD = Louis-James Davis, SP = Sarah Phelan and LD = Lynsey Dalglish.

KD: "I'm Kenny Dalglish, I'm going to be taking a rapid covid-19 test and the results will be uploaded to my V-Health Passport."

L-JD: "Sir Kenny will be taking his rapid covid-19 test and the results will be uploaded to the digital V-Health Passport."

SP: "Your hands there then please." (mumbled under a mask and 'welders' visor)

LD: "So, we're here today to do the rapid antigen and antibody test. The tests will show us if Kenny has had coronavirus in the past with the antibody test. That will be a blood prick test just in the tip of his finger and that will give us 10-minute results. The antigen test will tell us if he currently has covid and that will be a nasal swab test and those results will be in 15 minutes."

L-JD: "The V-Health passport is test agnostic. It can work with any form of test - the rapid test, antigen or PCR test."

SP: "Okay Kenny so both tests are over and your antibody test is negative and the antigen test is negative too."

KD: "Negative! That'll do me.

It's getting to a stage now where people are looking to take the next step, and the next step is to bring fans in - if it's at all safe. The first and most important priority is the safety of everybody. The more readily available your results are the better, and the more secure the app is, the better it is for the people coming in.

Sarah, if you can just send it to my V-Health Passport."

SP: "Yes."

KD: "Eh look! Look!

Hi, I'm Kenny Dalglish an ambassador for V-Health Passport... There you are - pretty ugly! Ha Ha. It serves its purpose. Ha Ha..."

The day after fireworks night, there was a different plot hatching, with the BBC weighing in with:

'Covid app backed by Zara and Mike Tindall prompts safety concern... The VHealth Passport allows Covid test results to be uploaded to a phone'.

It seems Mike and royal wife, Zara, were energetically, spookily, heavily promoting something for which, no doubt, they gave any fees to charity.

This would build, no doubt, on the NHS covid-19-84 app from Google. There's also an app, it just 'appens, shinily offered by Apple, as Snow White's friend looks on.

Days later, I received a near snow blizzard of emails from Louis-James when I trod on the frog that was an 'immunity' pass-port discussion.

Well, pray tell Einstein, just what does a test and digital proof enable... if not to go unmolested through the turnstiles of life, if it is not?

"I'm clean, I'm clean, I'm clean, Captain Peacock".

Inferred 'immunity', my little word sorcerer, that's what - despite the 'immunity' claim being a very hot as Tyndall on Kindle, hot button. As a flat frog looks on.

More horseshit and tram tickets, methinks.

There is also, natch, a neat and dandy (promoted by Randy Andy?) NHS QR Code, 'in case you or your loved ones have come into contact with coronavirus (COVID-19)'. Apparently, you can get an even cooler scanner to look up yer code. The scanner is so good, it can even track, trace and spot you from... Uranus. Which is precisely where I will stick it if some TikTok-time-bomb of an unhealthy munter from the NHS, waddles towards me - and tries to use it.

Speaking of more murky goings on, Elizabeth Hart, lord love her, has waged an almost one woman show against Rupert Murdoch, and his Wizard of Oz, tyranny 'down under'. They've been at it for decades, the Murdochs, with their own media empire.

Increasingly so since son, James Murdoch, signed up to the GSK corporate gravy train in 2009. More richly, under-served, he was pitched on to GSK's 'Corporate Responsibility Committee'. His dad has been deciding election outcomes for years.

But worse, their media empire covers up GSK's criminal vaccine harms. The $ky really is the limit for their ambition, with junior Murdoch setting an example of corporate irresponsibility, him being up to his axle stands in covering up GSK vaccine harms.

His doctoring protégé is no less than Dr Richard Freeman, the Team Sky cycling doctor. Who, in court, peddled 'the fact' that he destroyed a team laptop with a screwdriver... in an attempt he says, to protect the privacy of individual data... Just like

Pinocchio, he's clearly a puppeteer and a free man. But not at all free with the truth.

More locally, on the Isle of Man, Manx Radio has to get by on a £20,000 per week crowd-funded, taxpayers' subsidy. Come October 2020, the Manx treasury was doling out another £200,000 of crowd-funded budgetary provision numbers to them.

Might we be overly optimistic to expect the Cook Report style investigative digging into covid-19-84 pig troughery?

Reassuringly, the treasury quotes, 'this will be subject to the usual scrutiny and approval process prior to agreement'.

The mainstream media has, since when I was a kid, morphed sloth like into: lame-stream media. "Ah, lad - I remember reading The Express, back when you could buy a house for a shilling and the entire wages of Accrington Stanley were four bob for the year! Including their Brylcreem rations". I also remember when The Cook Report and World In Action, weren't what the media is now, simply a: whirrrrled-innnnaction-of-dissss-traction…

Pray tell, just what is the sex of the coronavirus, as Manx Radio have pondered?

I've been set up myself, on air. During one Manx Radio interview (on vaccine harms) I was lined up, bent over, and greased with the interviewer's words, "and some of his claims are controversial". Closet baby killer, brain reset from the get-go.

She, the baiter, is clearly happier than I am with bits of aborted tissues, metals, preservatives and pesticides being injected into the (coincidentally and controversially) sickest youngest generation ever. And later a bit of Abbotswood flu vaccine murder thrown in for good measure with 96% of them. But somewhat, researchedly and old-fashiondly, I am not.

The Manx Examiner is not known for baring its teeth - their controversial content quotient being a tad more Ken Dodd tickling stick than a 2am visit from Mad Frankie Fraser with a sharpened chain saw. A man whose 42 years in jail did little to smooth off his edges or blunt his blade.

But it seems the Freedom of Information request by the Manx Examiner was, er, examined and held to be too tabloid truthful so needed to be redacted - and some. If you can call 13.5 pages out of 15 a redaction - more like a blackwash with a thick dark pen. Add a bucket or two of creosote.

The redaction was related to covid-19-84, a truth that dare not speak its name; a topic that has had barely a column inch, or two this year. Perhaps as the topic was only of passing interest we, as a little rock in the Irish Sea, are not ready for truth-tellers. The response to the covid-iot 2020 plandemic was best kept secret under collective responsibility of the Manx CoMin (Council of Ministers) rules. Those rules being all for all and none for none.

The press have also made no mention that Stanley Johnson, father of Boris The Bojo, penned his book The Virus back in 1982. It's about, as if you can't guess, a virus and contagion afflicting the world, wreaking havoc and unleashing state control. They say art mirrors life - more likely, life mirrors the dark arts. And a timely, turd polishing script.

Media, the sands of time are piling up.

This has been quite a while in the coming. The 1993 film, Falling Down - starring Michael Douglas as a raging, tiny fused worker, who flipped his lid at everything and anything comes to mind. His racist scene in the Korean store was the stuff of infamous 'legend'. He would likely get the Asian mis-take but, in his rage and identity politics, he surely missed the CORONA ST sign, in plain sight.

As Jordan Peterson opines, 'We are now seeing the thrashing end of identity politics and compelled speech'. Quite. We love him although I don't get his meat only diet - but that's for another day.

So, for my uncompelled speechy friends Sum and Shitfur, please form an orderly queue as to who has the most: woke, leftie, con-servative, trans, gay, black, vegan, christian, jewish, atheist, straight, and muslim friends.

Short arses, puleeze, squeak up at the back - you Dutch fellas just stay where you are. Being a grey haired old coffin dodger, me sen, I'll attend (if not shadow banned) as a lapsed english, proudish, self-anointed representative of the walking, but early, dead.

I only hope I'll be allowed to express all my WPWB (White Privilege While Breathing) attitudes. Out loud. But… once we actually move on from labelling compelled speech and identity politics we might see each other without any tribal descriptor.

When we finally wake up from the energy wasted on the covid-con, we will, based on evidence, realise that:

We are all some dumb fcuk. Aren't we Dr. Ashford?

The increasing vaccine schedule mirrors the increase in The Silence of The Prams - and I heartily apologise if that term offends.

You can't have a talk about SIDS (Sudden Infant Death Syndrome) without mentioning the lion-hearted and calm words of Pathologist, Dr Waney Squier. One who follows where the evidence takes her.

Waney Squier has changed her mind; that her previous views on 'shaken baby' syndrome (syndrome = a posh word for we're not sure) were incorrect, based on the lack of evidence in support of the thesis (thesis being another posh word for 'we're even less sure'). No crash test dummy yet, nor acceleration monitoring device, can induce forces necessary to cause 'shaken baby' harm in young brains.

So, what else could be to blame?

That is the huge question, undermining all 'shaken baby' convictions.

The answer, of course, that few dare look at is: vaccines, inconveniently - while being the only product free of legal liability since 1985 - which in my mind is very convenient. Since which date the official US vaccine schedule has quadrupled.

Waney did a magnificent TED talk in Wandsworth and in 17 minutes highlights how we should all ask better questions that might yet shake accepted science to the core.

In my view SIDS is, often, Sudden Injected Death Syndrome.

I believe, if we care enough to look, we will find the evidence.

With US lockdown in March and April 2020, simple comparisons may show that with vaccine schedule disruption, there was a 30% reduction in SIDS deaths. The evidence will be easy to find - and there is no 'may' about it. The criminal purveyors, though, will use the well-worn, 'coincidentally'.

The 'covid' catastrophe is emerging as a slow moving iceberg, coming into view long after media mania has moved on.

Toxins investigator, Robert F Kennedy Jr has highlighted over decades the slow insidious harms of environmental and physical pollution. Now, the toll of mental health harms is becoming plain to see.

His figures are shocking, but can be mis-read, as to quote, 'one death is a tragedy, but a million deaths is a statistic'. He goes on to confirm that, in the US, for every 1% unemployment increase there will be an extra 37,000 deaths. Unemployment has increased in the US in some places by 30%. In May 2020 the official total was some 33 million. The final, on-going, toll from this insane covid-criminality will be more than a million suicides. In the US alone.

In the UK according to the NHS Mental Health data 168,000 more people sought help from NHS England for mental health problems in August 2020 as compared to August 2019.

It is also extremely disturbing to know that for children, the figure is 32,000 more in the same period.

1) Next   2) Skip   3) Ignore

During March 2020 everyone was at it, while walking slowly to a different drum. Fear was on the pre-schooling menu; for breakfast, dinner and tea.

1) New words   2) New distance   3) New normal

1) Repeat   2) Repeat   3) Repeat

The numbers are starting to come in, and what an earner (via the bankers) it is too. The Yanks are $2 trillion in the hole and up to their hubcaps, while the Brits limp along on the hard shoulder finding a mere £350 Billion for covid-itis. That would buy three years of NHS spend.

Matron, have we lost our collective minds? Yes, we have, and Matt Handcock is here to explain his wise spending. Although he did get a November white feather drubbing from Peers less Morgan for avoiding morning telly interviews for six months.

Also weighing in was Susannah Reid, Good Morning Britain's finest. Half way through the 20 minute extravaganza she implored handjob to just get testing as that's what the families want.

If John McGuinness spills his cornflakes over that public health bird from Edinburgh, think what he might make of thicko Susannah? She being criminally negligent to evangelise case-demics that will kill some of her viewers, the infirm and immune compromised, to boot. If I may verbally put it in.

I know the snowflakes won't like me calling her a thicko but it is the best word, and certainly most polite, I can think of. Do some bleedin' homework madam, or just leave the studio quietly. Or meet me on camera, in a court.

Unless you've been living with Elvis (and Lord Lucan) on the moon you've heard about 'covid' and/or coronavirus. They're fairly interchangeable terms; a bit like Tony Blair and war criminal.

With official UK government 'lockdown collateral' figures of 200,000 deaths 'covid' must be a bit serious. It must show: sky-rocketing deaths, provable autopsies, and be based on an identifiable virus. Failing all three tests, would be slightly embarrassing - as massive legal cases are now being flung about the world. Likely these multi-$/£/€-trillion claims have legs, real science and copious evidence to back them up.

Never, in our wildest dreamy nightmares (except for the 2012 London Olympic Games Opening Ceremony) did we imagine this year. Well, most didn't but some did; as they had The Plan.

Chinese; in recognition of their countrywide, mass mandated vaccination policy and the turning on of 5G in their first 'Internet of Things' city. Known incidentally, coincidentally and categorically as...

Wuhan.

Back in 2004 the French had signed an agreement with the Chinese to establish a joint highly infectious dis-ease research lab. Based, Dean-oh! like, in Wuhan, to 'weaponise' material by adding: 'gain of function', to bits for injection... The lab' was granted a highest level 'bio-hazard status' so it could knock up things... likely, even more hazardous than anything found in a Turkish wrestler's jock strap.

Two years later, in 2006, and the bird had truly flown, clear over the cuckoo's nest of insanity. Arriving on the well-greased palm of the media it was suddenly, drum roll, avian flu time.

But the marketing was all wrong, guys. Catch yerself on. Sadly, your 'H5N1 strapline' lacked any catchy, comforting tones or nice teeth of the covid-ring-of-confidence. But, at least, the narrative got a limp-wristed try out; one, when first floated, of lockdowns, lock-ups and lock-ins. The lockdown ideas of Richard Hatchett failed, mainly because his surname alone, buried him.

But, by 2020, and with better planning it's now finally fear. 'There is nothing so powerful as an idea whose time has come'.

How have we come this far? To advance about as far, Baldrick, as an asthmatic ant carrying two heavy bags of shopping.

Neil Ferguson, that's how.

Not content with being the 'guru' that sent over a million cattle to their deaths, he pulled another contagion wheeze with his covid-19-84 modelling predictions. The kind of modeller's map that even a three year old with blunt crayons could colour in better. Far better.

First it was 510,000 deaths; then it was less - about 95% less, to be roughly precise. But as no - repeat no - government has yet uniquely identified covid-5G, covid-21, or the earlier variant currently labelled covid-19, we should doubt the man in every way.

Especially when he, and shitty whitty, get pretty much all their dosh from Kill Gates. When you actually look into all their sordid affairs.

I know, you're thinking I can't say 'Kill'.

But that's what's happening.

Shall I move along, then?

Okay.

With us having lived (and continuing to do so) through the greatest 'pandemic' ever, should I mention the blatant disregard that Neil Ferguson had for the government imposed regulations put in place to protect us all, when he needed to ignore the lockdown in favour of going to see his lover?

Or should I not?

Twenty years ago, I used to troll up to Imperial College, and be impressed with the fancy buildings, but remained unaware of their corrupted morals. I used to invest in such early stage medical spinouts. Not so much invest, perhaps, but punt as the greedy spiv I was back then.

As for sage, we recall it is usually rolled out with onions on

Christmas day, for the stuffing. It used to signify an octogenarian sitting peacefully in the corner ready, but only if asked, to dispel deep knowledge. It used to define the wise. But SAGE when it has been capitalised? Well, what an utter pee take on wisdom.

The SAGE (Scientific Advisory Group for Emergencies) committee seems stuffed with conflicts of interest. On 16th March 2020 Neil Ferguson predicted 510,000 UK deaths from 'covid' and 2.2 million US deaths. Out of the 20 committee members 60% have received funding, or work for organisations from those who will benefit from a covid-19-84 vaccine. I wasn't allowed to mark my homework at school, but it was always brilliant.

There are four times as many modellers/statisticians on the committee than there are virologists. There are no immunologists nor nutritionists nor those who are paid to keep people well - and out of fear.

Ferguson has not had a great prediction record. In 2005 he predicted that up to 150 million could be killed from bird flu. In fact, slightly less died. The total number was actually 282 deaths. So, less in this case = 149,999,718.

Birdbrained people listen to Ferguson, who admitted that his 'covid' model was based on undocumented 13 year old code, intended to be used on an influenza pandemic rather than a coronavirus. Which is ironic, as on 8th October 2020, the NHS confirmed that in the post truth world all flu deaths would now be attributed as 'covid'.

Oh, and for good measure Ferguson refused to allow his code to be released for other scientists to check his results.

Can we jail all these people and soon? More so, as behind the 'covid' curtain, lurks the legal case with all the science printed in JAMA Paediatrics and Environmental Health Perspectives.

The mantra repeated ad nauseum that fluoride is, 'safe and effective' is now fully in the gutter - it is based on ignorance.

'Federal Court case to end water fluoridation.' People (apart from sleepy Joe) know that fluoride is a major toxin of the brain, and especially for developing foetuses.

Environmental toxicologist, Dr Paul Connett, cites fluoridealert.org and the evidence of wholesale Chinese exposure of children to heavy fluoridation. Compared with less fluoridated children their IQ is 20% lower. (Don't worry the aluminium nano-particles in the vaccines will do the rest).

The individual urine levels in mothers provide all the evidence from Canada and Mexico, if needed, as do 65 major studies confirming IQ harms.

Thank goodness the eco-educated spent six years fighting water fluoridation of our Manx water. Since they defeated Big Fluoride, there has been a trebling of fluoride harms studies.

I'm just saying that science, conflicts of interest and ego move at glacial speed. Remember that, when the unquestioning repeaters bang on with their 'covid' fear-porn.

And their final solution for the masses.

By 2012 the Americans were coming but all a bit big-hat-no-cattle as Harvard and Wuhan Universities started to do some (not-so-funny) monkey business. Note to Dr. Fauci: please stop knocking up in a lab poison particles for your four decades long vaccines.

Let's ask a medic...

Dr. Scott Jensen has form as a family physician, and not bad form either, in his 40 year medical career. That he is also a republican Senator for Chaska, put him in the verbal cross-hairs when he questioned the official 'covid' narrative. He took issue with the Centres for Disease Control (CDC) prevention policy citing that they were 'too squishy' and could artificially inflate case counts.

Maybe squishy translates into english as fraudulent?

Particularly when the CDC is not an agency, but a private for-profit corporation working for the United States of America, another corporation, doing lots of business in Washington DC, a city state with municipal thieves as well in it.

Criminal, criminal, criminal by: Fauci, Fauci, Fauci.

Three years later, but still five years ago, on 13th October 2015, it was eerily early but patently a good time in the land of prize guessers. I remind you of our Richard, of the Rothschild family. Not content with being minted, he thought it a capital idea to whack in an all cap's COVID-19 biometric smart-phone-generated, data Patent. COVID-19 named, shamed, ready and awaiting in the wings. Clearly Meg had lent Richard both her balls. And some polish.

In October 2019, The Plan was visibly being played out (except to those at the deaf, and mute, BBC) and hosted at The Johns Hopkins Center for Health Security.

This pre-planning event foretold a mass world contagion of a deadly 'virus'. The script and details were getting honed, but only amongst the insiders. They say you can't polish a turd, but you can roll it in glitter. The event was recorded for posterity so, if you find yourself bored anytime, you can view it online at your leisure. Just search for Event 201.

The Tempest was soon to be unleashed - then suddenly the BBC were granted a ring side seat and free tickets. But only if they started booing and hissing, at the ugly sister.

Obviously, one does not have to be a genius to guess who the main sponsors of that Event 201 were?

Well, the World Economic Forum and Bill and Melinda Gates Foundation were collaborators on the project too.

One might tire of me picking on Bill so, maybe, I should turn attention here instead to his wife, Melinda.

Of course, she generally doesn't get as bad a rap as her husband but when she wants Black people in the US to be one of the first to get the rushed (liability free) 'covid' vaccine - as higlighted in her interview during the virtual Forbes 400 Summit on Philanthropy back in June 2020 - I think it's fair to say: a racist and a eugenicist is a rare combination indeed.

Now, to be fair, she did say there are some 60 million healthcare workers (in the world) and they deserve to get the vaccine first.

But in the spirit of inclusiveness she also said many indigenous people, as well as people with underlying symptoms, and elderly people would follow after the Black people.

By November 2019 the wheels of Big Business were spinning and Mystic Meg was again plying her trade - what with all 50 US States advertising for employees offering exciting job opportunities as: 'Quarantine Officers'.

Ready, get $et... go.

The smokiest of smoking guns in this covid-con job was when

they banned autopsies. As if facts didn't matter to the post truth medics.

Recently, in 2020: car accidents = 'covid'; ventilator deaths = 'covid'; gunshot wounds = 'covid'; cancer = 'covid'; heart attacks = 'covid'; flu (most vaccinatedly of all) = 'covid'.

Welcome to the world of death by substitution. But no increase in numbers.

Some of my mates are in the Rotary and Lions club, even the odd piccie gets in our press here. The latest I've seen with a polio picture laments how we need more polio vaccines to:

1) stop   2) polio   3) sooner

or some such well meaning but banal chatter.

If only my mates on their million mouths marches realised the polio vaccine causes polio. When you look at the actual strain of the particles in the vaccine. But likely, you won't.

Stop using DDT and other pesticides in '3rd world countries', give them decent food and clean water; magically polio goes away.

Plus, India will stop seeing mass paralysis which Mr Gates has caused to 500,000 Indians.

It is deliberate.

Ah, yes, the multi-billionaire philanthropist who only has our welfare at heart.

Can we talk, though, about his population reduction TED video from 2010, that 95% of people and 99.9% of Rotarians and Lionistas, haven't yet seen? Is that okay?

To quote he, himself, Sir, His Loyal Holiness, His Royal Personage, High Priest of Baal (and Epstein Island Visitor) Mr Gates,

"Now the world today has 6.8 billion people, that's headed up to about 9 billion. Now, if we do a really great job on new vaccines, healthcare, reproductive health services, we could lower that perhaps by 10 or 15%".

This was transcribed from a video dated 10/10/10.

Plans take time.

He left off that he and his wife would target Africans first. He didn't get to be that rich without knowing where the diamonds were buried.

As an insider, when asked in January 2019 at Davos on CNBC, what was his best investment, he said investing in global health organizations aimed at increasing access to vaccines had created a 20-to-1 return.

Over the past two decades his Foundation has 'donated' "a bit more than $10 billion", and has created $200 Billion over those 20 years.

He's definitely a pretty shrewd guy and knows the 'business' of vaccines well.

Now, obviously, we must all trust everything Mr Gates says and does because of all those lovely $-billions he has. That alone is a good enough reason, isn't it? I mean, why else would we trust this man to look after our health?

He's not a doctor, he's not an epidemiologist, and he's not a virologist; although, in fairness, he does own vaccine companies, and he does own various patents. Oh, and he never

49

finished college and he's a documented thief. That's fine, then.

Dare I repeat, that non-doctor Gates said,

"Now the world today has 6.8 billion people, that's headed up to about 9 billion. Now, if we do a really great job on new vaccines, healthcare, reproductive health services, we could lower that perhaps by 10 or 15%".

So population reduction, however you look at, is definitely part of the plan whether the 'conspiracy theorist' label gets thrown around or not.

These 'theories' are heightened by what is sometimes referred to as the 'American Stonehenge,' the Georgia Guidestones which were completed on 22nd March 1980 (3/22). These towering slabs have inscriptions - supposedly the 10 commandments of the New World Order - which are written in 8 languages. In english they say:

1) maintain humanity under 500,000,000 in perpetual balance with nature.
2) guide reproduction wisely-improving fitness and diversity.
3) unite humanity with a living language.
4) rule passion-faith-tradition-and all things with tempered reason.
5) protect people and nations with fair laws and courts.
6) let all nations rule internally resolving external disputes in a world court.
7) avoid petty laws and useless officials.
8) balance personal rights with social duties.
9) prize truth-beauty-love-seeking harmony with the infinite.
10) be not a cancer on the earth-leave room for nature.

So along with reducing the world's population, helped along by the vaccine agenda, there's the side effect of there being money in it.

Likewise the covid-con is a significant money generator, for some, too.

Already, $100 billion has been allocated stateside in 2020 and to quote, '... and such sums as may be necessary for fiscal year 2021 during this emergency period'.

Please define 'emergency'?

Best guess, probably not, 'less deaths than the 2018 flu season'.

Since which time, coincidentally, flu deaths have fallen off a cliff, and FLU is now more simply spelled: COVID.

The Irish are great, love 'the craic' and over a pint or two, are fond of the saying, 'catch yerself on'. But we might not know, that is a joke, as... you-can't-catch-anything... scientifically, as Thomas S. Cowan, MD, and Sally Fallon Morell spell out in, The Contagion Myth - Why Viruses (including "Coronavirus") Are Not the Cause of Disease. In 300 pages of evidence.

But how so, oh shallow one, has the con-tagion-con conned u$ all?

Well $cience and proof$ of forgotten hi$tory that'$ how. For, as they say, 'If we don't learn from history we're con-signed to repeat it'.

It was John M Eyler who put the evidence together back in 1918; it was his, dare we say, 'war story'. His research paper was titled: The State of Science, Microbiology, and Vaccines Circa 1918; Public Health Reports - 2010 Supplement 3, Volume 125, p. 35.

'We entered the outbreak with a notion that we knew the cause of the disease, and were quite sure we knew how it was transmitted from person to person... if we have learned anything, it is that we are not quite sure what we know about the disease'.

"The research conducted at Angel Island and [similar experiments]... continued in early 1919 in Boston broadened this research... including a search for filter-passing agents, but it produced similar negative results. It seemed that what was acknowledged to be one of the most contagious of communicable diseases, could not be transferred under experimental conditions."

URGENT 999 and 111.

"Call the doctor, I didn't know I was ill but I've caught a bad dose of case-demic flu from Manx radio." The more we strive the more we stink. Test$, test$ and yet more test$. Myself, I just wish someone would knock me up, out of bed, and test me. I'm suffering from the poo, wee and sweat virus. The latter especially when I catch it from 9 otherwise healthy guys running around playing five-a-side footie.

In February 2020, satellite communication honchos, SES, launched a press release, confirming the Diamond Princess has 'the best WiFi at sea'. With too many 'covid' deaths onboard, though, suddenly it was bury the story time; as the ship was con-firmed 'in quarantine'. Get socially distanced from the press guys, pronto.

Make sure... the ambient environment changes, stress the cells, as wifi at 2.4GHz drives out water, while the 5G, at 60GHz, drives out oxygen. ER Doctor Cameron Kyle-Sidell please take an early bow, in New York for spotting the hypoxia, the blood oxygen issue, not the misdirected: 'covid-lung' claims.

So, you clots, it seems we're looking down the wrong end of the microscope. What starts out as a respiratory issue soon starts to be a blood and vascular one if, my little diamond princess, we look carefully. If it is a vascular disease then the best antiviral therapy is not an antiviral therapy.

This resolves a mystery of ventilators killing people - because doc's were treating the wrong causes and mis-reading the symptoms. Blood vessel damage would explain why people with high blood pressure and diabetes were susceptible.

On the 11th, the WHO were March-ing to a different drum, and declared covid-19 was a... pandemic.

The Brits weren't in lock-step, nor in lockdown at that time, as on 19th March, Public Health England announced that COVID-19 was 'no longer considered to be a highly contagious infectious disease (HCID)'- also, coincidentally, the day that the Coronavirus 'bill' 122, went before the UK parliament. At least Spielberg had a decent script and more animated puppets.

Four days after the non-HCID designation, and with less than four tenths of bugger all scrutiny, The Coronavirus Act 2020 passed on the nod, in the UK parliament.

The Emergency Bill was all of 358 pages and handy it was ready to be pulled out of the drawer. Ignoring all of Koch's postulates as the simplest proof that we, you, and Uncle Tom Cobley have been had - from behind - with a not so well greased cattle prod. To boot, Jack.

Worse than that, it's a Hitleresque 'Enabling Act' used, under the cover of 'protecting' people. If we imprison you, you'll be more able to be free.

Just two days later, on the 25th March - The Coronavirus Act 2020, received royal assent - which is a bit rough, as it was all ultra vires - beyond powers.

Or should that be an ultra 'virus' as it's: non-existent?

More like the dog that did not bark Sherlock - as there is nothing proven:

1) No Virus;   2) No Test;   3) No Contagion.

In just six words - that's it; just follow your nose, Watson.

During March it had been a gentle shimmy, but now into April out on the street all hell was breaking loose and people were doing odd things - performing a kind of latter day, military two step.

When out walking their dogs (along with granny and other botulism infested, coffin dodging, family detritus) people started diving into hedges, to 'get un-socially distanced'.

If that wasn't enough they clambered up lamp posts and scaled tall buildings with one leap, anything to get away from me, and my wife; her being, they clearly assumed, a fully modern day Typhoid Mary type. A, beyond the bizarre, experience.

I had other scary, covid-encounters of the 3rd kind... the most memorable occurred on a dangerous cliff edge. One Saturday, up close and personal trotted a Peel naturist - out no doubt for her daily Vit D top-up. She jogged nakedly, but distractedly, towards me on the very narrow path. I being, as ever, the gentleman didn't know whether to toss myself off, or push myself in...

Now that might be scary... but then there's a different level scary!

Of all the unbelievable b/s put out by the mainstream media

over the course of this scam, nothing I think comes close to being so hard-hitting, so scary or so terrifying as the report of Peter Sutcliffe being hospitalised with 'covid'.

Now, just think about it. Here's this 74 year old fella with a heart condition and one eye (no less) getting hospitalised with 'covid' and they report him as refusing to undergo any treatment for the 'virus' because he was 'terrorised' by it. And then he died.

So, you might be thinking what's wrong with that? 'Covid' is a killer so, having a pre-existing condition and in a susceptible age group, he should be terrorised by the thought of it.

Well, the story might be a little more believable were it not for the fact that our man Peter is a real killer - having the distinction of getting banged up 'for life' for the little matter of killing 13 (!) women (and attempting to kill another 7) in Yorkshire, England back in the late 1970s. Peter having been the 20th century incarnation of Jack the Ripper bludgeoning with a hammer, stabbing and disembowelling those poor women.

A genuine one-eyed monster for sure. Oh, and a mason, too, I believe.

A big red flag.

So, no, whoever dreamt up that storyline it doesn't pass the smell test... terrorised, my backside.

Talking of red flags the Isle of Man Courier proclaimed our island was subject to a 40 mph speed limit, to... 'ensure Noble's hospital does not become overwhelmed during the coronavirus pandemic'. I felt, oh so, relieved that being 10 times faster than the red flag days of 120 years ago. Progress - and empty Noble's wards too - if anyone with a memory asks.

Let's keep to the script that's been provided and just focus solely on the covid-con, please people! Well that's what our very own chief minister, Howard Quayle, tells tynwald (the Manx parliament) in late May 2020, "The era of the antibody test will soon be upon us".

Proving precisely what... in real terms? Pray explain.

An antibody confirms only a scene of a reaction; not protection, not history, nor predicts the future. He's clearly learned nothing from rampant disease-mongering to date.

Once Boris, across the water, caught the 'covid' it was only a matter of time until our Howard caught on too. Perhaps, it was when he turned on the telly that he realised how ill he was.

Long 'covid' but short brains.

Still in June, the Washington Examiner waded in with Maria Van Kerkhove, head of WHO's emerging disease and zoonosis unit, confirming that it's very rare for coronavirus to spread through asymptomatic carriers.

Someone should have asked, eff me boss, "How do you solve a problem like Maria?". Speaking off message, surely? Talking of which. They do like to use big words to make everything sound so important.

Like 'asymptomatic'. So scientific.

Asymptomatic is a bit like saying you're sick with the 'virus' but you're not actually sick with the 'virus'.

You what?

Exactly, you have no symptoms.

It's just the same as if you had no symptoms of the ordinary flu; no one would come up to you and say you were sick, would they?

Back speaking of the grand fromagers in central planning: The Council of the European Union document, 'Shaping Europe's Digital Future', in the Council Conclusions no less... buried down in item 36... spluttered out,

'EXPRESSES the importance of fighting against the spread of misinformation related to 5G networks, with special regard to false claims that such networks constitute a health threat or are linked to COVID-19'.

(or covid-5G as this author, will happily state as his statement of truth in common law).

On 19th November 2020 in an email to Gary Lamb, CEO of Manx Telecom I asked simply, if he would...

'Please confirm:

1. If Manx telecom has any 5G insurance?
2. If you, as CEO, have directors and officers insurance - both: a) in your employed role, and b) as a private individual.
3. The name and policy number of your corporate insurance.'

Because insurance will be of the utmost importance, in due course, when the 5G agenda is implemented here on our island.

I believe that 5G technology is not insurable anywhere on earth because its risks are unquantifiable. Go figure.

Now, Gary and I were once close.

In deference to Rudyard Kipling and his wonderful poem, IF:

'If all men count with you, but none too much.'

It pierces like an arrow, when truth is at stake.

You may be reminded of that film, Marathon Man, a magnificent thriller from '77 when the following interplay took place:

'Christian Szell:
Is it safe?... Is it safe?

Babe:
You're talking to me?

Christian Szell:
Is it safe?

Babe:
Is what safe?

Christian Szell:
Is it safe?

Babe:
I don't know what you mean. I can't tell you something's safe or not, unless I know specifically what you're talking about.

Christian Szell:
Is it safe?

Babe:
Tell me what the "it" refers to.

Christian Szell:
Is it safe?

Babe:
Yes, it's safe, it's very safe, it's so safe you wouldn't believe it.

Christian Szell:
Is it safe?

Babe:
No. It's not safe, it's... very dangerous, be careful.'

Meanwhile, still in EU heaven, even if the Romans didn't do much for us Monty, Milan's Covid-5G overlap map makes hot reading.

But one Roman who was roamin' in the gloaming, with an up early eye, was Dr Massimo Fioranelli. He has, on his own, gone not just speaking off-piste, but fully radioing in his warning. Being, as he is, from the Guglielmo Marconi University, in Italy and loudly chirping,

'5G causes 720 (factorial) different diseases in human beings and can kill everything that lives except some forms of microorganisms'.

Using the world 5G map, and over-laying with 'coronavirus cases' shows the picture.

Mid-summer and the balls sure are on the line, despite there being no footie.

That extremely well known corporation, Crisp Websites limited (trading as Pest Fix, with net assets of £18,047 and share capital of £901), hits a bulging net - when it netted itself, a pretty cool £108 million via a PPE UK Government contract.

Without so much as a, bye and you're leaving, tender process. Nothing wrong there. Nothing suspicious. Okay?

A somewhat delayed ref' may yet arrive and rule such a 'hand of god, golden goal' to be offside. A red card sending off, and time in the sin bin of mailbag sewing, may await. City AM has since reported that The Good Law Project has instituted a lawsuit. Spot the ball(s) up anyone?

This is not the only dodgy, under the table, dealing going on though. Remember, we're talking government 'dealings'.

A much more serious one is the contract awarded to Genpact (UK) Ltd in London who were awarded a contract without competition by:

the MHRA i.e. Medicines and Healthcare products Regulatory Agency.

The procurement description was:

'The MHRA urgently seeks an Artificial Intelligence (AI) software tool to process the expected high volume of Covid-19 vaccine Adverse Drug Reaction (ADRs) and ensure that no details from the ADRs' reaction text are missed.'

Part of the explanation given in the contract award notice 2020/5 207-506291 regarding lack of competition for the contract was:

'Strictly necessary - it is not possible to retrofit the MRHA's legacy systems to handle the volume of ADR's that will be generated by a Covid-19 vaccine. Therefore, if the MHRA does not implement the AI tool, it will be unable to process these ADRs effectively. This will hinder its ability to rapidly identify any potential safety issues with the Covid-19 vaccine and represents a direct threat to patient life and public health.'

So call me mad all you like, but I'd say that is a wake-up call right there.

I don't recollect seeing any mention of this little thing in the mainstream news. Maybe you have?

Now, if you're an accountant two plus two won't necessarily equal four but I hazard another of my guesses that this ties in perfectly with our friendly US $multi-billionaire, Mr Gates, wanting to vaccinate all 7 billion people against covid-19 (including those who have 'had' it).

In an interview on CNBC he said, "We have... you know... one in ten thousand side effects. That's... you know... way more. Seven hundred thousand... you know... people who will suffer from that."

Yes, I know; it's just numbers.

700,000 victims. Say it quickly.

So, that would also tie-in, nice and coincidentally, with his hope and wish from back in 2010, of reducing the population by 10% to 15%.

But let's not be unduly concerned, shall we?

Certainly he isn't; because, before the vaccine is actually given to the entire world he said, "... governments will have to be involved because there will be some risk and indemnification needed before that can be decided on".

Same playbook as always with the p-harm-a companies; indemnity for them all round. Profits only allowed.

Physical costs to be borne by those harmed through the covid-19 vaccines and any monetary costs to be borne by the governments i.e. crowd-funded from the people.

And, of course, you couldn't possibly blame Mr Gates himself could you? He's just doing all this because he's a 'philanthropist'.

The media, his politician friends and scientist friends certainly wouldn't blame him... for fear of having their funding cut.

I know I sound like a broken record but these people are criminals.

Included is David Ashford, our 'health' minister, who on 18th November 2020 in a media release on www.iomtoday.co.im said,

'We have been waiting and hoping for a vaccine for Covid-19. We need to ensure our population can benefit from the vaccine without undue delay, and that means having appropriate legislation in place. By bringing these amendments to Tynwald a month earlier than planned, we are keeping ahead of the game. Our clear aim is to establish a new protocol to allow vaccinations to go ahead at pace, safely.'

So, these amendments were planned anyway.

And, to be clear these amendments to the legislation are just to make sure the vaccines were safe for the island's residents?

Am I right? Well, not quite.

As he explained, it is to,

'...create immunity from civil liability for specified individuals (e.g. healthcare professionals) from any loss or damage that results from the use of a medicinal product with a temporary authorisation in accordance with a recommendation/

requirement that has been made by the MHRA'.

That's the same MHRA, by the way, who awarded that AI contract for the software tool, '... to process the expected high volume of Covid-19 vaccine Adverse Drug Reaction (ADRs)...'.

So, hang on a minute. Am I mad?

I don't see how this has anything to do with safety. It's all about covering one's ample anus from liability.

This is criminal in its intent. Lodge that, Lord Raglan.

So back in mid June 2020, another ball person is showing up with a sponge and half an orange to treat covid-itis. But the pitch has been queeried, so he's not being allowed on by the ref'. Just WHO's adamant that it is not a level field?

Junk Science, (great name guys!) trolled out, 'lawsuit alleges hydroxychloroquine kept from Americans'.

As an anti-malarial drug, it has proven safe, in the correct doses, for over 70 years. Only problem was that Trump, trumpeted, that it worked against (the, once mentioned) covid-itis.

But his enemies prefer a bit of death in, unhealthy, US people.

Unhealthy politics?

Meanwhile, conspiracy-realiters would cite that Gilead's touted Remdesivir is $4,000 / dose; while zinc, azithromycin and hydroxychloroquine combined, is less than tuppence-three-farthings. The fact the former doesn't work only adds fuel to the media manipulation $tory.

Soon the vaccine cavalry of AstraZeneca arrived but, being

cowboys, they wanted protection against the Indian peasants, who were revolting.

"This is a unique situation where we as a company simply cannot take the risk if in... four years the vaccine is showing side effects," Ruud Dobber, a member of Astra's senior executive team, told Reuters.

"In the contracts we have in place, we are asking for indemnification. For most countries it is acceptable to take that risk on their shoulders because it is in their national interest," he said, adding that Astra and regulators were making safety and tolerability a top priority. Along with a warpspeed vaccine, suitable for 7 Billion (unique) people.

Another call for indemnification?

Adds up. Back to bed.

By July 2020, we were going clean round the bend and, for once, finding myself in a pub, I unusually spotted Formula 1 on the wall mounted sell-a-vision. Most interestingly, the McLaren team all sported orange masks, adorned with 'we race as one', down in the pits... lane - hardly trumps a WWG1WGA slogan but near enough.

Next up Lewis Hamilton, in natty mask, as was every other bought and sold out plandemic communitarian billboard.

I was hoping the theatre would include his english be-masked-on-message-bulldog, but someone must have kicked his balls. On the lawn.

Meanwhile, Kary Mullis, of team PCR Testing Truth, didn't bother to qualify. He knew others were running low on bald tyres. He feared they would never get a grip, especially when the independent scrutineer showed up and the rains came in.

A dip-stick test would soon have the spectators coughing and spluttering over doctored fuel.

Summer was passing fast, while that august organ, the Isle of Man Examiner reported that the reply to their Freedom of Information request was mainly redacted:

'Cabinet Office keeps most of advice about Covid-19 secret. One document, dated 8th April 2020, had 13 and a half of its 15 pages completely redacted' it said.

Imagine if you bought a thick black pen and when you got it home 90% of it was missing - you'd ask for your money back. Can you do that when suffering from: covid-covert-condescending governments?

By 14th September 2020, the local 'health' minister, David Ashford, was going walkabout at a public meeting with the fine people of Ramsey.

Talking of walkabout I was hoping he'd bring Jenny Agutter with him - but no luck. Such a shame, as I'd enjoyed the soft touch of her nursing skills in BBC's, 'Call The Midwife'; while, amongst the other nuns, I'm not sure Jenny had the tightest wimple.

As the public arrived, some had been filling the void and crossing the chasm, as we'd handed out 'Covid Facts Not Fear' leaflets, for balance - although one flu vaccine pushing doctor (receiver of £10.19/shot, I may add) declined to take one. But then her earner, sorry surgery, in town to jab the old 'uns beckoned, and loomed-largesse-like in early October.

At kick off time, it's standing room only with around 100 locals, scarily unsocially distanced, packed into the town hall. Unmasked, too, with not a face nappy to be seen.

The 'covid' questions were fielded by a local news reporter but all seemed steered and orchestrated and, dare observers say, a bit dumbed down from the off.

More than a low-ball delivery, it was full under-arm time, with the obligatory, obsequious mass clap (but missing the mass debate) for the NHS. With empty wards and no mortality increase, when you verify the scientific and medical evidence for yourself - it was beyond me.

As the evening wore on, apart from pondering on:

What is the sound of one hand clapping?

I was mulling over ventilator-caused 'covid' deaths and under-employed coroners.

As soon as Mr Ashford mentioned the 'she', who invented the PCR 'covid-test', my blue fuse-paper was lit.

I stepped forward, unasked, and called out, "She is, or was... a he!"

Kary Mullis was actually a man but, sadly, now a deceased one, in the life of post truth facts.

Handy then that Kary died, coincidentally, in August 2019 before the corona/covid-19 scam could properly take off.

Yes, therefore, we can ignore him. Dead men tell no tales or can contradict the narrative.

"Scientists are doing an awful lot of damage to the world in the name of helping it. I don't mind attacking my own fraternity because I am ashamed of it."

Okay, I see. That's pretty clear what you're saying, Kary.

He was also filmed saying,

"I think misused PCR is not quite… I don't think you can misuse PCR, the results, the interpretation of it, if you can say… if they could find this virus in you at all, and with PCR if you do it well you can find almost anything in anybody - it starts making you believe in the sort of Buddhist notion that everything is contained in everything else, right? Because if you can amplify one single molecule up to something that you can really measure, which PCR can do, then there's just very few molecules that you can have at least one single one of them in your body, ok? So that could be thought of as a misuse of it - to claim that is meaningful. It is.

There's very little of what they call HIV, and what's been brought out here by Philpott, and - the measurement for it is not exact at all - it's not as good as measurement for things like apples. An apple is an apple, you can get something that's kind of like… if you've got enough things that look like an apple when you stick them all together you might think it looks like an apple. But an HIV is like that, these tests are all based on things that are invisible and the results are inferred.

PCR is separate from that process that's used to make a whole lot of something out of something, but it doesn't tell you that you're sick, and it doesn't tell you that the thing that you ended up with was gonna hurt you or anything like that".

As if that wouldn't be enough - and it wouldn't for many clearly - there is Judy Mikovits, author of 'Plague', who said in an article, Why PCR Testing Is a Bad Idea,

"We're taking a swab and scraping some epithelial cells [from the back of the sinuses or throat] because that's what coronaviruses infect… We get a little RNA… and then we amplify it [through a] polymerase chain reaction.

We're only taking a piece of the virus, we're not taking the whole virus… and when you amplify something a million times, or 10 million times - whatever they do in the 30 cycles or so - it's logarithmic that RNA then is way overestimated… [But] no [viral] particle was identified or isolated from your saliva or from your nasal passages. Nobody took the secretions from your nose or your mouth and isolated the [actual] viruses.

A PCR test can give you a lot of false positives [by amplifying RNA fragments].

A piece of nucleic acid is not a virus. And it's certainly not infectious."

Judy also recently wrote the best-selling book, 'Plague of Corruption'.

So, like I say:

1) No Virus;   2) No Test;   3) No Contagion.

Anyway, back to our public meeting in the local town hall. Despite 24 Manx (claimed) 'covid' deaths, the man from the ministry was paddling without a canoe, and map. The 100 attendees in Ramsey town hall, kept their own counsel.

With Kary, a Nobel Prize winner, having said that his PCR test should not be used as a diagnostic… quite why our 'health' minister, Mr Ashford, would call it a 'gold standard' is open to proper debate and scrutiny.

Reiner Fuellmich brought VW to its knees in court over falsified testing of their vehicles. He is now well-funded to expose the fake PCR test. That he has Robert F Kennedy Jr alongside, means vaccine truth will also be well aired.

The recent Portuguese appeal court ruling, whose decision was dated 11/11/2020, has just proved precisely that the PCR test is unsound 'legally'.

Please mull on that... as the covid-crime unfolds.

Gradually the tempo quickened and, with blue lights in the air, all of a sudden it was foxtrot oscar, if you catch the drift. My hot yoga teacher; yes her, yowled for the moon with an impassioned, "Wake the fcuk up!" to the assembled hordes. Followed by, if I recall correctly, "Fcukin wake up!" as to the real agenda(s) in play. The vicar nearly dropped both his jam scones.

Later, in front of those 100 people, I mentioned that the 20 deaths at Abbotswood nursing home were "medical murder", and not due to 'covid'.

Nature abhors a vacuum as does truth. In court.

Fortunately it was filmed (viewable on Manx Health Matters) because, as ever, all unrebutted lawful (or legal?) evidence stands as truth in law. Whereas, anything ill-egal is simply a sick bird.

My ask of the evening was that the Manx government provide evidence of their 'covid' claim, on which they based the decimation of countless lives and livelihoods on the Isle of Man.

The skeet (Manx gossip) is that government hired hands subsequently visited our media providers, instructing them to skip asking awkward questions, or as a yoga teacher might say, with care and compassion, to: STFU.

Therefore, we must examine the role the flu vaccine is playing in all this, as 120 days after the Fluzone flu vaccine is administered, the deaths are 6 per 1,000. The claimed death rate due to 'covid' is 2 per 1,000 (refer Robert F Kennedy Jr).

We must examine if it is actually the flu vaccine programme that kills.

This would be easy when you have medical friends conducting such trials, in Singapore. As I do.

Nursing home deaths account for 80% of the deaths across the world - we must examine the co-factors including nutritional status, lack of daylight and lack of human touch.

Unfortunately, this year's annual flu shot roll-out is not going so well. At least for the vaccine pushers.

On the 10th October 2020, in a land far away, The Korea Times reported:

'South Korea's health agency said Tuesday that a total of 101 people, most of whom were elderly, died after receiving seasonal flu vaccines.

The deaths had stoked public anxiety over the safety of such vaccines, but the Korea Disease Control and Prevention Agency (KDCA) said 97 of those deaths have very limited relation with the flu shots. Another four cases are under investigation.

Of the total, 84 people were aged over 70, followed by eight under 60 and nine in their 60s, the KDCA said.

The health authorities have repeatedly said they have found no direct link between flu shots and deaths, urging people to get flu vaccinations before the onset of winter amid the coronavirus pandemic.

Public anxiety has heightened over the safety of flu vaccines after some vaccine bottles — part of the country's free inoculation program — were exposed to room temperature during distribution. The authorities, however, said there was no safety issue.'.

Abbots wood say that, too, wouldn't they?

An Inspector doesn't call.

In all fairness, I will point out, though, that the CDC in the US have been quick to follow up on what is undoubtedly a serious scandal over there in South Korea.

The following is taken from their website:

'Deaths in South Korea Following Flu Vaccination

As of October 26, CDC is aware of media reports of 59 deaths in South Korea following flu vaccination with flu vaccines distributed in South Korea.

The Korea Disease Control and Prevention Agency (KDCA) reported that most of these deaths involved people in their 70s and 80s. The KDCA has investigated 46 of these deaths and has reported it did not find evidence of a causal association with flu vaccination. Autopsies were performed on most of these 46 people, and all had serious health conditions that could account for the cause of death. Of note, among the total deaths reported so far, there has been no association with anaphylactic shock, a serious allergic reaction that can follow immunization, according to the KDCA. The KDCA has not suspended its flu vaccination program and is continuing its investigation. CDC will continue to monitor this situation closely.'.

You will note the discrepancy of the CDC saying only 59 deaths in comparison to the 101 from the Korea Disease Control and Prevention Agency.

However, irrespective of which number is considered, isn't it strange that the CDC is quick to point out that, '... most of these deaths involved people in their 70s and 80s.' and in the 46 cases they investigated they are so certain that there was no, '... evidence of a causal association with flu vaccination. Autopsies were performed on most of these 46 people, and all had serious health conditions that could account for the cause of death.'

Oh, as an aside and to be clear, should a baby or child die within 72 hours of having any vaccine then, most definitely, the vaccine would not be responsible in such instance either.

Strange how they say that isn't it?

Now, for the covid-con they have a different approach; if someone dies from any cause within 60 days of having a positive PCR test that death is counted as a 'covid' death.

Old age and any serious health issues are clearly only a relevant factor in considering the cause of deaths when it comes to flu vaccines.

In covid-land all associations, connections and truth are inverted and perverted.

And, criminally corrupted.

Unlike my first book there are no links to be found at the rear of this one. With the unprecendented mass media censorship, digital book burning and broken-link returns having accelerated it would be a pointless endeavour. Far bettter, if you feel inclined to look deeper, to do your own research. Who knows what other serendipitous material you might find?

These words here are, after all, just the warm up act but what's unfolding is not jovial Ken Dodd - and most definitely not being steered by diddy men. But they do wear funny hats and clothes and speak in tongues.

So just how did these covid-nazi's get such power?

Planning and sleeping masses, for a long while, that's how. A bit like Mussolini, I suppose, at one time the most powerful man in Italy; but his gig didn't end too rosily did it, Benito?

You see what most people don't realise is that nothing is happening 'by pure chance'.

The majority of us usually go about our daily lives without too much concern or foresight for the future. True, perhaps, many are concerned when the next payday is and we may be looking forward to next year's holiday - yes, well, good luck with that one!

The travel industry has been decimated through this scam; many smaller companies have already been forced to close, and others are currently limping along after seeing business cut by 90%-95%. (We'll conveniently overlook those big companies with close connections to governments and who have been recipients of billions of $, £ and € bailout money, crowd-funded from hapless taxpayers and unlikely ever to be repaid.)

Anyway, planning...

One man few would have heard about before 'covid' came on the scene is a chap called Klaus Schwab. He was the founder of the World Economic Forum (WEF) and also created the Forum of Young Global Leaders back in 2004, whose aim was to help the world meet increasingly complex and interdependent problems. All very laudable.

No coincidence that among its members have been the likes of: David de Rothschild; Alexander Soros; Mark Zuckerberg and Emmanuel Macron. Other well known names include: Tulsi Gabbard; Daniel Crenshaw; Nico Rosberg; Rio Ferdinand and Amal Clooney. Nice.

The Plan is laid out in the 2010 Rockefeller Global Levels of Control document. We might also wonder at the 2015 COVID-19 Patent, and the lucky guessing distribution (in 2017/2018) of the 'covid' testing kits…

What foresight.

In 2019, too, another patent was lodged by the queen's golden shared Pirbright Institute, assisted by Serco.

But the grandest of all plans Blofeld, is the multilevel, multi-connected WEF - looking towards achieving a New World Order; as Bush senior warned ominously on film,

"… and we will." some 30 years ago.

This is all about a planned reset. But you didn't write it.

They want to schtick a Schwab up your nose; but let's first pause.

You may have thought that 'covid' is the only game in town... But you'd be wrong.

On 8th July 2020 Schwab said, "We all know, but still pay insufficient attention to the frightening scenario of a comprehensive cyber attack which would bring to a complete halt the power supply, transportation, hospital services, our society as a whole. The COVID-19 crisis would be seen in this respect as a small disturbance in comparison to a major cyberattack.

To use the COVID19 crisis as a timely opportunity to reflect on the lessons the cybersecurity community can draw and improve our unpreparedness for a potential cyber-pandemic."

So, don't say you haven't been warned. Never mind the coming covid-21, they're setting us up for the cyber-pandemic, too. You never know, they may yet pull out the 'alien' card, too.

Pandemic has a certain ring to it, though, don't you agree? A frightening ring to it. Be afraid. Be very afraid.

They have to tell us; that is their 'code of ethics'.

Some people may have a predeliction for youngsters while others might get their kicks through their nazi-like tendencies.

Schwab up your nose, throat and anus (best in that sequence, too). Is there a patent on that shitty schtick?

Born in 1938 in Ravensburg in Germany, Schwab was a child in the time of Adolf Hitler.

The Nuremberg Trials that followed the war were a series of 13 trials carried out between 1945 and 1949 to try those accused of nazi war crimes, and so Schwab would have turned nein(!) during that period.

Have no fear, the New Nuremberg Trials are coming.

At least in WWI the shelling stopped for footie on Christmas day. Penalty and football. That lot thought they'd get away with it, too; that there would be no penalty in extra time.

We can learn from Simon Wiesenthal, who spent much of his life hunting down those who thought they were above the law in the carnage of WWII. How public sentiment changes when people wake up from a dream that turns into a nightmare.

More so, when Simon authored the template of true service to your fellow man. His book Justice, Not Vengeance shows how the 'covid' criminality will unfold - as the many wake up, demanding that justice be done and seen to be done.

They: Klaus, Tony, George, Barack, Hillary, Nancy and their ilk think they're untouchable. You do that when your entitlement and expectancy traits harden. When you're deep in smug alley, eating the canapés with Davos man. Many of those further down the food chain also have that false sense of security, believing they're protected from their actions.

Wrong.

Close to 400,000 survivors of the Holocaust are believed to still be alive today. One of those, Vera Sharav, is the founder and president of the Alliance for Human Research Protection (AHRP). She is a public advocate for the rights of medical research subjects in the US. As a result of the draconian measures undertaken in the US during the 'covid pandemic' she has given a strong warning that if people do not stop blindly obeying authority, the U.S. will very soon be just like Nazi Germany. And not just the US.

Anyway, back to the planning... and predictive programming. You may remember the London Olympics opening ceremony, back in 2012, had the dark and dystopian NHS scene with symbolised scary 'covid' catchers. Operation safety-pin, and Paper Clip, in one.

We were subsequently to discover, in mid 2019, even queen madge, young Madonna, had some kind of affinity for the eclectic. The image on the cover insert of her new CD showed a corona-brand typewriter.

And, she appeared in the 2019 Eurovision song contest wearing a crown (corona) and an eyepatch. Quite naturally.

Her whole performance during the show was fully symbolic and ritualistic. During part of it she ominously intoned,

"Not everyone is coming to the future;
Not everyone is learning from the past;
Not everyone can come into the future;
Not everyone that's here is gonna last."

I know, I know, it's just entertainment.

Tom Hanks has been in on the act, too - down under. For this, though, he only had a supporting role. On 11th March 2020 (11/3) he let his fans know that his wife and him had caught the 'covid'. Fortunately they survived.

But with the news the mainstream media were able to dig deep and we were blessed to get a glimpse in to the collecting habits of the rich and famous. How fascinating to find out that he was a connoisseur of vintage typewriters... and his all-time favourite was one from the corona-brand.

We also got a look behind the scenes at how kind, thoughtful and generous a man he is when the media told us that Tom had sent a letter and a corona-brand typewriter from his treasured collection to an Australian boy. A little boy. The boy had taken the time to write to Tom about being bullied over his own name: Corona...

Clearly the makeup artist has been working overtime behind the scenes.

Track and trace and test and trace are the details, the mere trickle down, obedience, tactics. You don't get to see or vote on the $trategy. You never do, that's why it feels so alien and why you feel so out of sorts.

It's deliberate.

Self-Isolating is a new term, jolly trendy and up-selling it is in a glamping-on-the-moors type way.

Measures enforced across the world have seen the imposition of 'covid' martial law and quarantine. These have caused untold harms to lives and livelihoods so these science-based measures require full and open scrutiny. Evidence must be considered.

However, everything would fall apart for them and their paymasters if:

true science were examined;
true evidence was presented;
true deaths were autopsied;
true numbers were compared;
true causes were identified;
true lessons were learned.

Not being given the opportunity to do so in a true court, on and for the record, is criminal.

They will not even debate.

What would they be afraid of?

They are quick, however, to jump and label any questioning of it all as conspiracy theories and when that doesn't seem to work they use the all-time favourite last-resort of calling you an anti-semite.

I had that offensive label thrown at me in May 2019, before this covid-con, when simply presenting one of my self-researched notes, that contained 182 links to articles, peer reviewed research papers and videos to back up what I was saying.

One of those 182 links included the word 'Israel' in its title and that alone gave enough cause for the good doctor Allinson to throw that slur at me - wrongly assuming I would run away and cower in the corner.

No such luck Alex.

Oh, and if I'm not wrong, I think Noah was called a conspiracy theorist back in his day, too...

And then it started to rain.

Robert Koch defined such evidence to verify that viruses can actually cause any specific disease(s). These four requirements are known as Koch's postulates and are requirements for any 'virus' claims.

Postulate 1: The parasite (virus) must be present in every case of the disease.

Postulate 2: The parasite should be fully isolated from the body and all products of the disease, i.e. purified.

Postulate 3: The parasite should be grown in a pure culture (this is not possible for a culture to be pure).

Postulate 4: The isolated parasite produces the same disease with all of its characteristics in a normal host.

To date this 'novel' virus has only been cultivated in transgenic mice, infused with an ACE2 gene (that mice don't normally have) to 'prove' the possible infectivity in… men and women. In the end the results of causation weren't statistically relevant, just some mice with 'slightly bristled fur' - to quote.

This is Frankenscience, not the expected evidence to shut down the Isle of Man, or the world, is it?

The Centers for Disease Control and Prevention have had a slight covid-cause rethink. They've rolled back 94% of all those they claimed to have died from 'covid'. When the department of justice started looking at the numbers into ho$pital fraud, suddenly the death tally figures went (miraculously) down from 150,000 deaths to 9,000.

My word. An error in the cooked books of 141,000 deaths, who the media had mis-spoken about hourly, and daily; but weakly it seems.

That an (untempting?) $13,000 was reimbursed for each registered 'covid' death may have encouraged wrong accounting book entries - not just double dipping but double counting.

Careless whispers, costs lives, George.

There is a new novel RNA vaccine on the blocks… £100 billion on testing, aiming for 10 million tests/day. In the blueridge mountains of Virginia health commissioner, Dr Norman Oliver, has just stated he will mandate a 'Covid-19' vaccine. He won't be alone…

Medical practices which start out in the US normally arrive here two years later.

The only product with liability exemption is the vaccine.

First enacted as law by Ronald Reagan in 1985 due to the likelihood of pending claims due to bankrupt the highly profitable US vaccine industry.

The US vaccine injury compensation fund has paid more than $4 billion in harms compensation, despite only 1 in 100 harms claims being reported, according to the Harvard Pilgrim Study.

These 'legal' claims are held in private, without any process of discovery, 'courts' before 'special masters'.

Anyway, back on 13th October 2016 PC (pre 'covid') I had the head honcho guys behind VCode® and now V-Health Passport, VST Enterprises, in my lounge. If you've forgotten already, they are the storm troopers behind the passport of purity endorsed by Sir Kenny Dalglish.

Those, whose crazy diktats now decree which festering pieces of infected humanity are allowed to travel. Freely, unmolested, from Health-Row airport, formerly known as duty free in Heathrow. Best stay out of the death-row, if you've nothing to declare.

What a crap shoot of stupidity. To use a useless test for a non existent virus, to say who can and can't travel to their holiday home, or to attend granny's must-get-to funeral. This is not gonna end well, if I can avoid speaking in (v)code.

This Manx registered company doubtless seemed like a wizard wheeze when the founder had his unique identifier tattooed on his wrist.

But, having been to Auschwitz on my motorbike, I was quite different when riding home. Seeing photographic evidence of pitiable people tattooed in such camps, changed me for ever. How can that lesson be missed and glossed over?

Or where new 'technologies' will lead?

If any of this is true, then it is mal-feasance in public office for which individuals will be held liable in their private individual capacity.

If our man, Klaus, gets his way the fourth industrial revolution is planned to be the biggest yet - by 2030.

The previous revolutions, we note, upended at least one table and spilt some milk - if history is any guide. But this time it will be different. It's a technological race to trans-humanism, where the individual is obsolete and up on bricks.

Klaus spells it out in more detail in, Shaping the Future of the Fourth Industrial Revolution:

'Fourth Industrial Revolution technologies will not stop at becoming part of the physical world around us—they will become part of us. Indeed, some of us already feel that our smartphones have become an extension of ourselves. Today's external devices - from wearable computers to virtual reality headsets -will almost certainly become implantable in our bodies and brains. Exoskeletons and prosthetics will increase our physical power, while advances in neurotechnology enhance our cognitive abilities. We will become better able to manipulate our own genes, and those of our children. These developments raise profound questions: Where do we draw the line between human and machine? What does it mean to be human?'

That's what Klaus thinks anyway, commanded by his overlords.

Even the disgustingly evil S.S. 'officer' Klaus Barbie could not have dreamed in his wildest nightmare what his present day namesake, Klaus Schwab is lining up.

Barbie was known as the 'Butcher of Lyon' for having personally tortured prisoners of the Gestapo - primarily Jews and members of the French Resistance.

While Klaus was busy torturing, staff of the Bayer group at I.G. Farben were busy conducting medical experiments on inmates of the concentration-camp at Auschwitz.

I.G. Farben the chemical and pharmaceutical conglomerate has morphed over the years, and today goes by the name Bayer-Monsanto.

Once the authorities had a change of heart they put on the Nuremberg trials and directors of I.G. Farben were held to account. So, their suits (and silk ties) did not protect them after all.

The Nuremberg trials took a while to set up, so we applaud what is happening currently for 'covid' justice in: Germany, England, South Africa, Scotland, Ireland, Australia and the Republic of Kanata, formerly known as Canada.

Since 1918, 'Spanish' flu experiments were unable to show that flu spreads; it is merely a detoxifying excretion, inner or externally, triggered. The mass vaccinations and radio wave pollution were the causes back then.

We really must study Dr Stefan Lanka and Dr Antoine Beauchamp who are right; the terrain is everything - Pasteur's germ theory is no-thing. But our friend Louis sure knew how to get fake ideas to market.

As an aside, anyone with a PhD in Spanish Flu bolloxology and contagion please feel free to challenge me on camera under penalty of perjury.

No change there, then.

Rinse and repeat.

Spin cycle.

Bearing in mind the 'pandemic', as highlighted by the mainstream media, there is an equal feeding frenzy on Mother Teresaesque drug companies looking to save us. There were

236 vaccines in development at the last count.

In fastest qualifier position is Moderna - and were, for a while, the bookies' favourite having, of course, never ever developed a vaccine. This in an industry that takes, on average, 10 years to bring to market; however with the money - sorry lives - involved they can magik-ly knock one out in less than a year.

Better still it won't be the normal 96% failure rate seen in vaccine developments. Best go figure, Dr Dastardly.

But, solving the Joker riddle, the clue is in their name Moderna; as in Mode-RNA. It contains something extra for the boys and something extra for the girls. I'm not sure what's in it for the trans people.

It'll highjack your RNA, and forever re-write your genetic code.

Their stated aim is trans-humanism. Klaus will be pleased.

But Dr Mengele's brother has now rocked up at GSK, who are lining up 'one vaxx for him' and an equally 'special' one for her. None of this metro-sexual same vaxx stuff.

The girls get anti-HCG (first chanced upon when I looked at the depopulation, sorry the tet-anus vaccination programme in Kenya).

The boys get a different shot; a dose of GnHR. Game over in the beautiful baby stakes - but needs to occur so that the real Agenda 2030 'goals' can be met.

You don't have to be Agatha Christie to know that the lines will be changed, from the land of Poirot - as Belgium is where GSK knock out two million doses of vaccines... per day.

Now, on the railside, Pfizer is the dark horse going in to this dark winter. Handily dropping the news of a '90% success' rate with theirs.

Would it be unsporting of me to mention that, coincidentally, on the day of Pfizer's latest vaccine news which, naturally, boosted its share price in the market (no, not the wet fish or bat market, silly one, the share market) its CEO handily sold another batch worth $5.6 million... pump and dump, baby!

Don't be so quick, though. Within the week, one Prof. Uğur Şahin, BioNTech co-founder, the co-developers of Pfizer's vaccine was featured on BBC's Andrew Marr show. In the interview he said, 'I'm very confident that transmission between people will be reduced by such a highly effective vaccine - maybe not 90% but 50% - but we should not forget that even that could result in a dramatic reduction of the pandemic spread'.

Fair enough...

90% down to 50%; still fairly good, wouldn't you say? Because, in the narrative for us all, we'll conveniently ignore the fact that our own natural immune systems have a 99.9% success in working against the 'virus' to stop us dying.

In this upside down, inverted perverted world 50% (or 90% even) is better than 99.9%. Madness.

Your assistance in pushing this criminal 'covid' narrative marrs my soul, Andrew.

And about the speed of bringing the vaccine to 'market', that isn't really a problem, either, is it?

I mean, the testing for its safety is top-notch, right?

Maybe...

'Study to Describe the Safety, Tolerability, Immunogenicity, and Efficacy of RNA Vaccine Candidates Against COVID-19 in Healthy Individuals'

This study was posted to the US government National Library of Medicine on 20th March 2020.

Its official title is:

A PHASE 1/2/3, PLACEBO-CONTROLLED, RANDOMIZED, OBSERVER-BLIND, DOSE-FINDING STUDY TO EVALUATE THE SAFETY, TOLERABILITY, IMMUNOGENICITY, AND EFFICACY OF SARS-COV-2 RNA VACCINE CANDIDATES AGAINST COVID-19 IN HEALTHY INDIVIDUALS

Actual Study Start Date Z : April 29, 2020
Estimated Primary Completion Date Z : June 13, 2021
Estimated Study Completion Date Z : December 11, 2022

Or maybe not.

The fact that this study they're in the process of undertaking not ending until 11th December 2022 - so, in two years time - is not a concern?

Who are going to be the real guinea pigs in all this?

Well, on 17th November, 2020, Bloomberg.com published an article addressing a similar point across the pond:

'Vaccine Safety to Remain Unclear Until Millions Get Their Shots'.

In the piece they say, 'Vaccines have generally been safe, though some high profile missteps have helped fuel scepticism. For example, in 1976, some people who received a swine flu vaccine developed Guillain-Barre Syndrome, a might have changed on my route. Because, at the end of the day it's not only midnight, it's business.

But also before items one to three, I'd spent several thousands of hours doing independent research and seen the sick and legal businesses up close.

Including... reading hundreds of 'peer reviewed', but independent, medical papers. And most recently building a collection of legal books.

Much of the medical research was carried out when consulting for five years to the Isle of Man government, as a healthcare innovation advisor.

Medicine and law were not what I'd thought.

It was quickly clear that the men in black don't seem to like it when you turn up with a well batteried torch, to the institutions of state Halloween party.

I'd also been listening very regularly to John Farnham's wake up call, You're The Voice - and the line, "We're not gonna sit in silence" stirred something in me. With over 20 million views on Youtube, I gathered I wasn't alone - but nor was plod, as I was about to find out.

On Friday 12th July 2019, a week after my first arrest, it was blues but no twos on the Snaefell Mountain Road.

For six months I had been almost full-time researching common law. Wondering how I'd managed to miss true title to my property.

Not the pis-direction of watery owner-ship, as in a maritime sense, nor in the 'possession is nine tenths' sense, either; but full-on enjoyment of 100% of my property.

In case you're wondering what the last tenth is, it's the legalese trap. It's the paper bit. That matters, and it's theirs.

I'd decided to try out the theory on my conveyance. It was formerly a grey Renault Clio, registered number DN57 AYA; but most recently it was identifying as CLC JURBY. Especially when I'd changed the plates and more importantly I'd listed it under common law, and de-listed it with the DVLA.

To remain acting in honour - a key common law tenet - I insured it from the 2nd July 2019 with Manx Cover, receiving an insurance certificate stating CLC JURBY on it.

My arrest ten days later (and subsequent £600 fine for 'no' insurance) seemed not only a little rich but a lot: unlawful.

It's probably why the arresting officer, Stephen Hall, subsequently perjured himself.

Oh dear, and they say 'porridge is a revenge best eaten cold'. He was also the first, in my 62 years, to suggest I needed mental help. But he was the one unable to answer even the most basic questions of law.

My 'car' - my conveyance - has not been seen since Stephen, or one of his colleagues at police headquarters, stole it; when whoever it was dishonestly appropriated my property, formed the intention and took it upon themselves to permanently deprive me of it.

So, for now, force of law is winning. For now...

But a kindly police employee has since located and returned my CLC JURBY letter plates, a year after their theft.

Ironically, around the time of plate retrieval, my 12 months no claims bonus confirmation for the insurance on CLC JURBY duly arrived. Followed by Robin Blackford, of Blackford's brokers, trying to criminally coerce me into regis-tering my conveyance with the queen and her DVLA commercial enterprise.

Remember, she owns, you maintain - being bait and switched and 'required', in one document, to become the very down-market, 'registered' keeper.

If the police manage to get you into the 'driver' and 'vehicle' language trap then you are acting in 'commerce'. For their limited company that is then game on, joinder, and contract time. Sod that ma'am, you can foxtrot oscar.

Another year on and it was almost like groundhog day.

Monday 6th July 2020 I left home at 8.50am having packed my yellow vest, spare socks, and some sarnies. Finally, at Ballacraine crossroads a local MHK (Manx House of Keys) member turned right for the be-wigged, invitees and I turned left for the free strollers and free thinkers.

I arrived at Union Mills and at 9.30am, met my mate Lee - a 99% er, and donned our yellow vests; his plain and unwritten, mine with 'HPV VACCINE DEATHS' printed boldly on it - the same garb as on tynwald day 2019.

Little did I know, that I was heading for another tynwald day arrest in similar plod ignor-ance, but this time with an added spell in jail. For those who don't know, tynwald day is the day of doleance and petition for redress on the Isle of Man.

How quaintly ironic we're allowed such by government. In theory.

Another theory is that if people were told their brain was an Apple app, would they more willingly use it?

An hour later, after a nice stroll, we arrived at Ballacraine crossroads, 400 yards short of the 'official' tynwald day ceremony. We stood there and many cars passed. Some gave us long glances, and even a thumbs up from the odd MHK, and MLC - which, to be honest, was heartening.

We decided to stand away from the 'official' activities so as not to invite trouble. Or get arrested.

After another hour, the gentry were starting to leave - but not Trevor Cowin, whose eight petitions of doleance had been kicked not just into the long grass, but also into the swampy grasslands of deepest tynwaldia.

That today was our national day of enshrined grievance airing for all, struck us as rather odd - clearly we lacked the ability to define all.

Time marched on as cars sped off. I saluted the attorney general as he drove jagtastically by, as he but not I was doubtless on, official maritime rules, duty. Somehow, all the comings and goings on, just didn't seem like cricket.

I'd had better interactions with the attorney general during my five years as a healthcare innovation consultant to the Manx government, when he was onside with natural botanicals; but which five years on, had failed to take root, being as they are less toxic than all p-harm-a had to offer.

I've never understood the medical industry rinse and repeat model of sickness treatment - you'd think it was only done because there was money in $ick.

Last year the clerk of tynwald had also tampered with the ball, bowling earlier at my googlies by back-dating my petition. Perhaps hoping that I wouldn't spot a year's date change. Time travel could catch on with him - by pen. What's the legalese and Latin for git?

We soon took photos, alongside a 'road closed' sign - which aptly summarised the Manx government's blindness and deafness to the Manx vaccine-injured HPV recipients, and to those in other countries. With the regular bleating about being the oldest parliament, I thought they'd welcome truthful free speech.

With Black Lives Matter demonstrations sweeping the world, 'I took the knee for HPV', for people of all colours killed and maimed by this - the increasingly evidenced - most toxic of all vaccines. For 16 years evidence that Black boys suffer 3.4x the autism of white boys post MMR vaccine has also been ignored. Let's unite in knowing that it truly is a whitewash whatever the shade.

Police man Matt arrived around noon; an (unlawful) high noon by him, as it turned out. We shook hands; me as a gentle man he as a (likely unbeknown to him) road pirate, trespasser and forcible kidnapper. Next, with an open hands gesture he said, "You should know there is a warrant (war-rant) out for your arrest - my colleagues will be along to arrest you shortly".

He asked if there was anyone at home who could pay even part of the fine, hoping to get a financial instrument, and contract underway - so that I'd move along out of full view, no doubt. I genuinely believe he was trying to be helpful.

I said nothing, just gesturing to the 'HPV VACCINE DEATHS' yellow vest I had on, which may have mysteriously contributed to all things 'force of law' of their war-rant.

Alternatively, and plausibly, the serving of such a warrant seems to have taken exactly eleven months to the day, since I was last in 'court' - as the ink dries slower on an island in the Irish Sea.

Mentally, I dismissed his offers of business, joinder and entrapment - but I could see it wasn't cutting any ice.

"No", I replied, followed by, "it's not lawful and I'm not paying it".

Paying a fine for my 'non' insured Renault Clio conveyance, when Manx Cover had banked my money and issued a Certificate of Insurance for CLC JURBY, jarred with me. After a year passed I even received a one year's no claims bonus insurance confirmation for CLC JURBY, my non DVLA registered conveyance.

The warrant, supposedly, was from the Douglas 'court' case of 6th August 2019, demanding £1,450 to be paid within 28 days (that was the 'with menaces' part). Serving it nearly a year after the lapsed date, and arresting me on a second tynwald day in 2020 was pure coincidence.

As the boys in black had also previously been round to my home, trying to conduct other business, it can't have been because they didn't know where I lived - can it? A whip round for a crowd-funded sat nav' (or parchment map) had a certain appeal.

I explained to Matt that he had no authority nor jurisdiction, and nor did I consent. This fake land grab, abusing maritime law, via parliamentary overreach - a body we the people invented - has no teeth. Only brute force - and a lot of ignorance - which, as they are fond of telling us, is no defence in 'law'.

For that which we invented cannot rule us.

Our employees know no better, their assumptions and presumptions give them an untouchable air.

Backed by force of law. For now.

At least Matt, with a kindly smile, said he 'knew' not to call me "MR HEADING", so maybe he had done a tiny bit of research but skipped the difficult bits.

Note to self: free (new) book for Matt.

He's a nice chap, though, and (although hearsay) he tells me his mum wears a 5G protective pendant; she most likely could teach him much. (Like the 5G overlay map with covid-itis coincidence.) Then before too long, perhaps, he'll say "Gawd Houston, we really do have a problem", followed by "If I ignore common law, will it go away?". Nope.

If a tree falls in a forest, and no one sees it - is it still a man's fault?

After plod reinforcement road pirates arrived I handed my Common Law Court I.D. card to Lee. I also handed him my HPV yellow vest and, I believe, he had the common decency to stand in it for another 4 hours for the passing motorists to observe.

Then I was off, in a free van ride to Jurby, accompanied by Paddy and Pam. Paddy assured me he'd drive like a granny and he did indeed. I had already started to wonder if his granny was 1960's Pat Moss Carlson or perhaps the 1980's fire breathing Ur Quattro maestress, the fabulous French, and usually frighteningly airborne, Michèle Mouton.

Finally, on all four wheels, we arrived at Jurby at around 1.30pm; with no watch and no phone, time and fun had passed me by. We were met at the entrance to the prison by another two-wheeled road pirate (not Matt) and he had arrived with the case notes.

One thing I didn't know at the time, which apparently has worked in other cases, is asking if anyone present can identify the living man - as in me, as in 'courtenay'. Of the clan :heading.

The accused can't self-incriminate, so two witnesses would be needed on a summons. The police paperwork is just hearsay, whose similarity to the word heresy is worth a study on its own.

Obviously, I bring plod nothing but pleasure, so probably should get 10% reduction on my ransom fee. As Pam handled the notes she asked me about the case. I said it was unlawful so I wouldn't be paying any fine.

She seemed to perk up, "Oh, so 70 days in jail it is". Funny how some get their pleasure even when they seem normal-ish. Friendly criminal coercion, though, is still criminal coercion.

Ploddess Pam was interested in health apparently and said she'd look at my Jurby Wellness blog, free it was, and she was open to open thinking, as a bonus.

Lessons are useful, if we treat them as a reflective learning experience. Although, I'm guessing as I've not yet enjoyed a jolly good tasering, which might interrupt clarity of thought.

But for a personal 2021 vision, I reckon we'll again be highlighting the HPV vaccine crime. It's not going away, so nor will I.

If the covid-19-84 vaccine doesn't make people infertile, then fear not young satan, the HPV vaccine has already been engaged to do the job. It's quite simple. Women not HPV vaccinated have more kids. A simple comparison will prove that. So that won't be done anytime soon, except it might well be in summonses.

This is merely a ramble through what I've learned since more fully waking up to 'legals' around two years ago. I'd had many nudges over the previous 20 years but was too busy doing busy-ness.

As the law can be dull, I hope the odd bit of levity lightens the hours. With three arrests and two short jail spells I've tried to remain upbeat so that we can defeat this tyranny.

Now, by first serving notices of obligation on our public servants - who criminally transgress their oaths of office - we can.

As an example, together with two witnesses, I served an initial notice of obligation (including substantial evidence of treason, vaccine and 5G harms) on Gary Roberts doing business as chief constable at his place of business on 20th October 2020.

Having allowed sufficient time for Gary to do his own investigations, on Wednesday 18th November 2020 I served, together with a witness, a notice to compel performance on Gary.

These notices are part of the serving on 47 people in their private individual capacity while doing business as chief constable. This has taken place throughout the British Isles.

Fortunately, I was not arrested; unlike the Lancashire three, who were stopped on a motorway while travelling in their conveyance to also do a similar service. Coincidentally, somehow in advance, the policy men appeared to know of their plans.

If we challenge the 'vires' - the assumed legitimacy - in, say, a local magistrates' court, we should be asking for the case suspension, by calling for an up a level, judicial review. Let's not allow them to pick our pockets by paying any force of law, 'covid' fine.

If we don't get a suspension of any claim on us, we need to send it upstairs to a higher 'crown court'. Let the jury decide - being 12 good men, or women, and true.

If we overturn a 'covid' fine as being ultra vires, then an enormous legal challenge would happen across Britain, resonating elsewhere too; and that would paralyse the courts. Educating them for their over-stepping and dare we say, goose-stepping, is part of our role. We, too, were once asleep.

We should cite Boddington's - the law case, not the drink - as in 1995, Boddington v British Transport Police we have proper precedent. This was a proven case of state over-reach of them acting ultra vires. Let's drink to that and stand firm.

Never fear, in court terms, it is best to go upstream, into a superior court. For there, the air (and water) is less polluted. Plus, if you get swept downstream you're more likely to be carried away with things, and away from the lawful source.

Arguing over the little things, while missing the big picture is never the best place to be.

I'd been following Cal Washington of InPower Movement for a good while and loved his calm demeanour even when talking about the horrors that he and his brother had suffered at the hands (and batons) of the US police. Yet, he still remained philosophical, stoical and in honour. Impressive too that he is a clear communicator, as well as being optimistic and fearless.

He often said that, "If you go to court you've already lost", as good a warning sign and wake-up call as I could get.

As John Smith, of Common Law Court, also says, "It's best not to play in their sandpit".

However, my latest learning opportunity, is drawing me into a legal Manx sandpit.

My curiosity, in November 2020, may yet get me slicing my shot into the bunker of the 13th hole - to see if someone really has left an unsightly dog's egg in it?

But we must remember that any lower order Rottweilers, in a magistrates' court, can leave costly teeth marks. But if we don't face their fangs, we'll never know.

So we'll record the action.

Curiosity not only killed the cat, I also know that canine ways can land us in the dog house.

A long while back, at school, my friend and I were bored in art classes so he, for some reason, proceeded to poke the teacher's pet dachshund in the ear with the (rubber) end of a pencil. On the (un)lucky third attempt the dog bit him, to which Geoff - ever the shining wit, exclaimed, "Your dog bit me sir!". Adding, for effect "Unprovoked". Which was just a tiny bit rich, Pinocchio; but might have been recanted when he got caned. He suffered for his art.

So, noted, I have been duly warned about not poking dogs - well, only when per-mutted. But it's not all dark and dismal if we know our standing in the school of life.

In paddling around, if we stay upstream in their courts we avoid reductionist, siloed, costly to us, thinking.

First up we can then ask them, respectfully, if they are actually playing their necro-mancy joker card - exposing it, then trumping it.

This necro-mancy of theirs, is the language of the dead; their hidden in plain view, bewigged language. While dressed in black.

Their clues, for us, are everywhere and chivvy us constantly - if we awaken. But if we stay there, resolutely in their courtly sandpit, not belligerently, nor controversially, then the legalers can at times, melt away.

These legalers, are the people formally called: lawyers.

They do legal, we do law - and the two terms are most definitely very different.

We might ask them, respectfully, "Can the living accuser place their hand on the living accused?".

Will the bit of paper move towards you?

They, the legalers, only have force of 'law' left.

Quite simply, all that takes place in a current style 'court' is the pantomime of: living men walking - but dead men talking.

Their business in court is carried out 'corp(s)orationally' using only business to business language. Of-the-dead, but made verbal by you.

Too much isn't it?

How was I - for six decades - such a 'legal' zombie?

But you, as the living man or woman can't be dragged in there; unless, of course, it is done to you unwittingly.

Dead simple.

When you finally get your head around the massiveness, the

utter enormity, of this elephantine deception.

Have you got that?

The lawsuit, the paper, is the 'court' - shouty, shouty.

Worse still, I'm told, the paper size, can trip you up too; foolscap confirms common law, and A4 is for the legalese guys and girls.

The name on the paper represents your 'legal fiction' created at birth - your dead 'strawman'.

The combination of given name (creditor) and family 'surname' (debtor) are a trick, used to egg you into 'claiming' something that isn't you - the living man with mind, mouth and soul.

Every document that a legaler lays before you can be a trap, for the unwary and unwitting.

Trust documents may slip in such words as 'inter vivos' meaning throughout life - so trustees may end up grabbing the assets if that clause is not spotted, and you snuff it - without telling your next of kin where you've buried the family silver, on paper.

It's a classic Latin based: property bait and switch - but not one taught in my secondary modern/comprehensive school of the 1970's.

It's said that x marks the spot - but when 'x' is in a mortgage box it has already been signed, but by countersigning it you then assume 'their' debt.

The 'behind the curtain' dwellers have relied upon legalese perversion and spell-ings for centuries of entrapment words

121

such as:

person, citizen, liberty, register, worship, gifted, warning, and 'peon', as hidden in plain sight on pass-ports.

Common law eliminates word-smithery deception with transparently honest language.

By removing legal trickery we create a true living individual, one returning as an in-charge custodian. On land or in cyberspace.

I was six decades asleep, so I'm throwing no stones.

I've seen the goings on of family courts… what a misnomer they are. They make the nazis seem pink and fluffy in comparison. I'd never had dealings with them until 2020 and then it was suddenly a Hollywood horror show, to be a tiny bit honest.

What a baptism of fire I had, when helping a lady try to protect her born property, her young offspring - who others wanted to vaccinate. We soon stopped calling 'it' - her three year old - as we all tend to do… a 'child', otherwise you'll trip 'well' into the Baal, goaty worshipful guys phonetics, as 'killed' is actually the pronunciation of 'child'. No one's kidding, are they Tom?

The occult, the hidden, is unseen and the ultimate in word trippery - and it is a bit dark, to be honest. But that is not for now; this is just a primer. All you can do is warn those you wish to help and, if they don't listen, move on so you can help others on their journey to waking up.

I used to push too hard; more fool me. But always be on guard, so when a policeman cautions you… keep schtum and calm, and always park your ego.

We were taking on the 'family courts' pretty much in (g)utter ignorance and mostly, sadly, we were like a candle in a howling wind.

I recall when Fathers for Freedom were atop buildings with pleas written on bed sheets - likely because their partners had fully buggered off (with the much needed washing powder) and taking the spaniel with them, to boot.

Now, close up and impersonal, I was beginning to get how countless mums and dads always called each, once loved, 'the other side'.

But, truth be told, each side was being played.

The judge was the referee, dressed appropriately in black, and was being paid for, unwittingly, by the beleaguered. In the not so dry dock. Kept apart and distracted by the 'courts of common purpose' - whose aim is to become a surrogate parent.

The clear role of the state is nothing less than a legalese initiated relationship, insertion of an adversary - in a place of commercial business mis-called the: 'family' courts.

'Common purpose' being, as it is, a charity sounds so warm and cuddly, like friendly fire, or 'short of the ideal'. Sorry, I misspoke BoJo. It's obviously about us all working together, for the common good using common sense and where everyone wins. Always.

Just like the 'common market' was told and sold to us. By that effin' traitorous Teddy-Bare-Heath. Anyway, what if others are now at it, in hollowing out the old, normal… ?

So what if 'common purpose' is not all that it seems, allowing below par peeps, to leg one over on us, unseen? To slither and slide themselves into every aspect of our lives, while talking a very good race. Being wedded as they are to a caring, sharing, communitarian agenda.

Let's go all official, in case I've given them too bad a rap, more so as 'common purpose' manages to spew out several thousand alumni each year. From their website (commonpurpose.org):

'Common Purpose delivers leadership programmes in over 100 cities worldwide. We believe leaders who cross boundaries make cities work better: and cities that work better will be better at dealing with their own problems, and the world's.'

Brian Gerrish is a former naval officer - one who wears a tie almost all the time, so he isn't your normal anti-establishment rock thrower. Over many years he's highlighted all the 'common purpose' antics, and how they've inveigled themselves into every aspect of public life. But there are others who lurk, generally unseen, within public utilities, the government and, of course, the police.

A Freedom of Information request normally identies the subterfuge.

In studying their ways Brian sees their footsteps in the courts and judiciary especially inserting themselves into guardian-ship roles in families. Think corporate, profitable, communism as their role model. Obviously, they have the usual feigned obsession of equality, climate change, and screaming 'til their lungs burst, 'rights'.

Those 'rights', of course, protected the open-all-hours baby abattoirs during 'covid' lockdowns for other non-essential business transactions.

(refer p. 57 herein for the relevant numbers.)

If they say, it's 'your body your choice' when it comes to matters of abortion for women (and, being inclusive, men?), then why isn't it, 'my body my choice', in regard to other medical matters, my old pal Pol?

Natural common law states you must not force a proven, sharp pointed, deadly weapon - otherwise called a vaccine - on another. Just as you must not force any individual to smoke or drink.

It is beyond insanity that we tolerate this in Manx schools and beyond.

Anyway, back to my direct experience of the 'family court'...

At first it had all gone swimmingly or so we thought. Getting our ducks and paperwork lined up. A few days before the online 'court' hearing 'operation location' was put into force, and the passports of the mother and her offspring were removed.

Initially my friend was not keen to let her unannounced visitors in, as without a war-rant they had no 'write' of entry - spell-ings are all as many, too, are phonetics. But with an imminent threat to break the door down, and with a three year old in tears, mum acquiesced.

The next 48 hours were a period of homework, of avoidance of legalese, and boning up on common law. And sleepless nights.

Now mum, although bright, calm, loving and resolute was struggling. Everything - the stakes involved - was taking a big toll. And she was paying it. But me being, unwittingly, insensitive during that week asked, "How are you doing?" but I didn't expect her to start crying, over Zoom. Blimey. Big, big, stakes, if I didn't know that already. I had jude sit in on some of the calls to give that connection - that woman to woman vote of solidarity - a massive, over the airwaves, hug. When not much else would do.

The Zoom case started and mum was alone against the state and saying her piece, respectfully. Sometimes when she raised an awkward point they would mute her.

That's justice.

After the case ended she was told they would be in touch. They quickly set another case just two and a half hours later.

Not only would the ruling be that her daughter must be vaccinated, also when the estranged partner is in attendance, but she was handed down £-thousands worth of costs too. Tough times.

What we'd missed - in error - was that possession was nine tenths; the other tenth was the state-enacted fraud from birth via the capitalized 'birth' certificate.

Something that we are all counselled to not use for id-entity purposes; especially since 2016, when their plans expanded for the entrapping ID2020.

With this knowledge, though, we can make amends for the error by the process of:

1) presenting our requirement;
2) escalting to our demand;
3) seeking remedy; and finally
4) obtaining cure.

As an example on such a journey to obtaining cure, the

following notice of requirement was served in Sweden:

'notice to agent is notice to principal and notice to principal is notice to agent

notice of lawful objection

I sharon-may: of the family: israelsson: mcloughlin do confirm this is my statement. It is my lawful objection to your behaviour. I only present it in writing while I sharon-may am willing forthwith to give it voice to you Lena face to face. By your refusal Lena to make yourself available to receive my statement you Lena act in dishonour individually and in your business activities as chief alderman.

You Lena doing business as: chief alderman of: Sundbybergsvagen 5 171 73 Solna, Stockholm, Sweden are hereby required to cease and desist your actions and activities against me sharon-may immediately. The use by you Lena of any hidden constructive trusts in commerce will not be tolerated and these activities leave you Lena liable in your private individual capacity. I sharon-may am sure you Lena understand this don't you Lena? You Lena are required to stop your black art activities which rely on legalese a false language known only to Advokat members of the private Swedish BAR Association to which I sharon-may am not a member. I require all evidence be heard but not as currently in a selective lower private court.

There is clear evidence that I sharon-may have been unlawfully converted since my berth date by the use of criminal trespass. This was undertaken via my strawman an invented personation by others using my legal fiction. I sharon-may am in the process of establishing dominion over this deceptive legal fiction of this so called capitalised name. This name and surname trespass relied upon fraud ab initio as being fully without my consent and via deception upon my parents for profit. The remedy for this deception has no time limit. I am sure that you Lena understand there is evidence of this over centuries by liable individuals using deceptive corporations of business and maritime courts.

I confirm as a living woman that I sharon-may act souly within common law: causing no harm nor loss while being in peace and acting in honour at all times. I sharon-may am the true beneficiary of my life trust account despite others trying to usurp my lawful benefit. This criminal trickery has also been undertaken on my living property. Such property is my young man known as theodore :mcloughlin israelsson and my young man vincent :mcloughlin israelsson and my young woman known as lily-rose :mcloughlin israelsson. They are all mine to honourably protect and enjoy without interference. Any attempt by you Lena to criminally coerce me sharon-may or any attempt at guardianship by the courts upon my property will be rebutted under the strongest lawful terms.

I sharon-may will not be attending your place of business other than to verbally present this statement and I sharon-may will be accompanied by the witness kent-rune-krister named on page 2. Any failure by you Lena to cease and desist will be met with substantial claims for damages from me sharon-may and also claims from my properties upon you Lena. Such claims are not protected by your professional insurance due to deception and malfeasance in public office in this case ab initio by the creation of a constructive trust but one which was hidden from me sharon-may ab initio.

The activities to date rely upon force of legalese and deception passed off as law. It is clear that you Lena do not write nor speak in plain language however, I sharon-may, do. You Lena rely upon dog-latin false words of legal deception marginal text and inconsistent styles. I further require that you cease using manual of styles writing and legalese trickery in your words. We can only communicate in true english. I'm working with common law advocates so we may all remain in honour and peace.

I sharon-may and my property enjoy unalienable rights from our born date which no one can infringe without causing harm or loss. If there is no victim there is no crime while universal law is a true jurisdiction. You Lena will know that ignorance of true law is no defence. I sharon-may look forward to your reply within 10 days confirming that you Lena will cease and desist your fraudulent activities. I sharon-may present this true statement without malice ill will frivolity or vexation.

autographed

by sharon-may :of the family :israelsson :mcloughlin
          this day…………………………………………

Witnessed on and for the record

autographed

by kent-rune-krister :of the family :lagerquist
          this day…………………………………………

[Assisted by courtenay-adam-lawrence :of the family :heading

Author of: From Health Heretic To Common Law Advocate

Forthcoming book due out on 1st December 2020: The Covid Con; A Wake]'

~~~

This notice has been included with the kind and willing permission of sharon-may.

At this present moment the lady doing business as chief alderman continues to be obstructive in the process. Another mis-take of a myopic legaler. This is really tough; as it is de-si(g)ned to be.

Amongst the legalers, sitting atop the heap are judges.

Judges are normally former QCs (or silks), so no one blows the whistle on those remaining inside the tent. Those who they used to sleep cosily with. It's one big club.

Women more than anything in court, in the dock, don't get justice.

A lady involved in a £-multi-billion claim, put up an online petition and 500 women signed it within 48 hours. There is a tidal wave of injustice harming both sexes.

This particular lady has created many a video, some with Thames Valley Police and Crime Commissioner Anthony Stansfeld, who wholeheartedly agrees that both the judicial and banking systems are institutionally corrupt. The lady clearly states the courts have been weaponised, "my husband murdered and they, in the system, have bankrupted me - taking control of my estate".

This includes 'top' law firms and insolvency practitioners, engaging in massive asset stripping.

Anthony Stansfeld also affirms, "You're meant to be confused, there is a mingling of lawful and the unlawful - so you assume that you're doing wrong".

It's very much once you've grown accustomed to lies, the truth becomes a conspiracy. In reality.

Ah, reality; now then, now then, now then!

What if the judges are merely financially-driven administrators in an administrative hearing... and spell-ing?

What if Bill Turner is indeed right that: the paper is the 'court'?

And they never try living men and women.

At birth you are made the debtor by the surname; the name you are given is the creditor. We have a creditor account listed with Fidelity.com containing as it does, a portion of the mineral land rights of our birth land.

There is much to explore and I, too, am on a journey.

When I was a lad, drinking weak and warm beer in pubs, I often heard "last orders", so we knew we just about had time to line up three halves (of Harvey's bitter) and, if lucky, another pickled egg before the landlord threw us out at closing time.

The land-lord, no less - now there's a term and a half, but I was all at sea then, too, so didn't notice him.

Then, steadily, it was telly time for the voters, and we started seeing our 'leaders' in the televised British parlay-ment. And what a spectacle it was. Betty Boothroyd, the daughter of textile workers, was holding court back then, splendidly.

But later, the role was tarnished by the short-fused, and some say more short-arsed, John Bercow, the former 'mr speaker'. Now there is a new fella, elected in November 2019, Lindsay Hoyle, who somewhat less flamboyantly confirmed that, "The culture of bullying is now over".

Whoever could he have been alluding to? It's likely that Berk-Cow, had he squared up to anyone in my old skool would have got a right pasting after metal work. Behind the bike shed. While standing on his own stool, the little turd. Yes him. Un-parlay-ment-ary language, indeed! But not, perhaps, my honourable ladies and gentlemen, entirely without merit.

Anyway - he was only following orders, steering such a ship of state, as he was.

So, what has this to do with, "order, order, order" as is so often said in Westminster. Seat of her maj's government. Yes, note, hers - not yours.

It all comes from 'orders' - the taker and the giver. But orders should only followed by those, in certain roles, who agree to follow them - usually military types; and orders should not be issued upon the unwitting, without their informed consent.

Education is needed, as to what really are 'orders'.

When PC plod/ploddess signs on to uphold the law, they are, from the get go, agreeing to follow orders. Pretty much without question, although that is a wrong assumption. They believe:

1) they stand under the orders of their superior officer(s)
2) they believe and trust that numbers, called a fee, a certain number, will appear in their bank each month; as in sal-ary, based in Roman times as 'sal' or salt - the 'money' being salted away.

It's much the same with all official service personnel and private corporations.

An order, is something that we place on Amazon (if we want to support the poor, down and out, Jeff Bezos) and he fires off his drone with a payload of popcorn, plus the Eyes of Darkness by Dean Koontz, from his Wuhan bookstore.

When we order anything we expect to pay an acceptable amount in an acceptable timeframe for acceptable goods.

When we pay, the agreement becomes a contract. They set the amount and, unless we negotiate the price, we pony up, without a trap - or free manure.

This is a simple error because the price displayed by the merchant is not their offer to sell the goods at that price, it is only their 'invitation to treat'. You make the offer by tendering currency. The currency we use today is fiat i.e. 'by decree'.

Anyone who services an order is chargeable and the individual who carries out the order can charge for it. You can't expect it for free. If you try and obtain service for free that's an unlawful demand, and if you send several of your six foot three inch brothers round to ensure compliance at 11pm - that's a demand with menaces.

Or just as likely a call from the police. With whom you did not have a contract. Such an enforced act is trespass, and official people carry it out all the time.

For clarity, it is also criminal - no matter what posh frock they are in.

White collar crime is rampant, with mortgages topping the list.

They have so normalised, so institutionalised the criminal, but more of that later.

As you get entangled in all this one-sided football match, of deception, you can start to level the pitch, to tip it back in your direction.

Not only are they charging by the minute, the guinea brigade have a fee schedule; you can have one too. Your remedy and redress for their guinea foul.

Yes, when you cite your fee schedule that too is an offer to contract. You have turned the tables, on a level playing field. My yoga teacher would say, you have finally decided to stand in your own power. Simple.

Does your 'official' or your legaler work for free? Or the attack dog from the other side, or the bailiff?

No. Then neither do you, now.

It is your creative energy that they are seeking to hiddenly harvest. Not heavenly harvest.

A promissory note, which some call currency, is creative energy (or current-see if we relate that money is energy, re-presented). We know that currency is cash flow, which we take to a (river) bank, if we're liquid, in funds.

It's all water terms and maritime contracts when we look.

Water you waiting for, to cash in on - to this language? Who had the best navy in the world? The Brits, and they sure left their legal mark. Not just marks, they also stole dollars, pesos, shillings and much else.

That was back when money was 'real money'. In truth, few today understand what money is. This, despite the fact that people work themselves silly chasing it.

If you ask most people what money is, few will answer that it is just a belief system. A true con-fidence game. Get a few bits of paper bung a bit of ink on it, a few 'security' features, add a bird wearing a corona (in Spanish) and you're off to the royal races. I'm only half joking. Today, some even believe 'Bitcoin' is money.

Over the years many things have been considered as money including salt, shells and beads, and paper notes. None of these have ever lasted long.

The two things that have, though, are gold and silver.

'Gold is money. Everything else is credit.'
J.P. Morgan

'Let me issue and control a nation's money and I care not who writes the laws.'
Mayer Amschel Rothschild

and, from one of his sons,

'Who controls the issuance of money controls the government!'
Nathan Mayer Rothschild

The families who control the function of banking and lend the dosh to 'governments' everywhere, basically use magik to create untold amounts of wealth for themselves out of nothing.

At least they have birth certificates to guarantee their lending. Peon.

This wizard wheeze has been going on for quite a long while, behind the curtain Dorothy...

From time immemorial the bankers have always gotten what they want.

We had the run around the block in 2008, when the bankers in Britain got bailed out at a cost of £500 billion, by the hapless taxpayer. From the mass of crowd-funders, yet again.

In US at that time they hit the crowd-funders for $700 billion...

The bailout (maritime term) of our currency was decided upon by the same private schooled johnnies who rule us now. Pass the gold-plated baton and the bolly, please. Jolly good show!

Iceland had the right idea afterwards, gaoling for general delivery, the bankers. Keeping the cells warm.

Nowadays, the governments' paper promissory notes are becoming ever more worthless. The current economic model has massive levels of never-can-be-repaid debt. It can never be repaid (by design) because of the interest handbrake. More invented debt comes with interest. But it's not in our interests, nor our solvency.

That's what the great currency reset will usher in. With central bank issued digital currencies not dirty old cash - which the 'covid' nasty is devilishly attracted to. Unlike the cardboard packaging used to ship all your online purchases to you.

How many times can you be lied to if you do not know the truth?

Signed, sealed, delivered is a three word chant. A document needs to be all three to have correct standing.

Signs are where major frauds start, in short, where some become quids in... as the si(g)n changes everything. A sign can be anything that re-presents something.

An autograph is the writing that you auto generate in

confirmation that you acknowledge something, you give it your blessing - that it is in order.

The signs that we miss are everywhere, and usually there is money, deception and a power switch going on.

The blue fiver (British five pound note) had two bars through the libra sign, meanwhile the green fiver has just one. In plain sight.

The queen and her minions, are on the payroll. She only does this because they love us.

Not, mischievously, because she needs the extra fivers to help Randy Andy pay for another legaler - to get him off yet another 'you're kidding me' charge.

I think it is important to mention here a little about our British history; which others have done a far better job of describing so I'll present just a potted mouth version.

Way back in 1213 the Barons went to King John, as their open top sewers were not as good as his open top carriage. They were not pleased, so put wet quill pen to parched paper. Even then, rather than unsheathe the beast and have it all kick off, they wrote him a long letter.

After two years they still hadn't got resolution, so in June 1215, off they trotted to Runnymede where King John autographed the Magna Carta, and sealed it too. The basic aim to get the King in check. Mate. He, King John, was in service to we the people - to whom the Barons had sworn free allegiance. As our upholders.

This is the primary document which has forever set out our unalienable freedoms which no one can take away. It is a - without fear nor favour - proclamation.

A bit like when you get married, but without the fear.

These unalienable (unalterable) enshrined freedoms would later morph into the watered down claims for 'civil rights', a well meaning trap of privileges, obligations and 'benefits' - meted out to the 'worthy'.

In that term they switch you from the land of the private on shore, to the watered maritime courts of the public. But only if the cap fits and you sign on the dotted. They literally, militarily salute your ignor-ance of what is going on. As they pipe you aboard the good ship HMS Tosser.

As time went on there followed lots of acts of parliament, a place where they literally go to speak, to parlay to the mind, as in parlay-mental.

Fast forward to the 14th Century, and the church-iferous Pope Boniface now was at it, with his Unam Sanctum declaration, claiming the souls of all people on earth.

Cheeky sod, if we dig a bit deeper. And more than a bit rich, which is why the church is so... well, rich. Such, dare we say, one sided documents were called papal bulls. And we know what a bull does. In the woods, along with the bears.

Pretty soon after, in 1320, the Scots were staking their claim with the Declaration of Arbroath - doubtless signed somewhere smokie.

Then the gematria starts to kick in with numbers and symbols getting an airing. The scribes, of course, are often in on the secret but sometimes not.

The all-seeing eye atop the US dollar is still missed by many.

Top table, top of the pyramid, but you're not invited...

Unless you're a master mason, knocking up pyramids (which no one on earth still can... even if we give them, the secret ones, the 33rd). But that is a conundrum for another day. I guarantee I would be black balled.

So 1666 duly turned up, and it, more than any other year, turned us over. In our graves. Apparently, in London, it all got a bit hot at the bakers and the odd wooden house was subject to the far less happy: scorched earth policy. People died, and their families, dis-located.

So, sensing a jolly wizard wheeze, up pops some dangerous Latin sorts and devilishly, in 1666, the Cestui Que Vie act was born.

Latino man, however, forgot to tell us that. Absentmindedly. And we've been paying for his scumduggery ever since. We, the unwashed peasants, were suddenly all presumed dead. But at least we had (free, to peasants) open sewers to bathe in. If the rats hadn't used up all the soap.

So, in 1666 the origins of personation had arrived.

Someone, a churchy interloper, had inserted themselves into us.

Worse still, they wanted us to pay for their privileges.

Even more worse still, later, they talked posh and sneered as only slave masters can.

When you finally get the gist of all this, please tell me if my words have been a little cruel. Or lacking in respect.

The names of the criminals appear at different points in this book and, as for deception, the queen (one lizard of Victoria) tops the list. For theft.

Her (un-common) wealth was knocked off from the 'common wealth'. Of the mis-directed and distracted.

And, again, 1666 was the grand theft auto.

Auto means 'self' in Latin.

By pronouncing us all dead, and claiming the 'self, via our id-entity hijack we became slaves.

The Cestui Que Vie was a trust act, but we shouldn't have trusted them to act in our honour.

Ever.

Because they simply lumped the 'dead' souls and all of our creative resources forever under churchly owner-ship. There we go, another maritime ship sails in to us, HMS Rectum, later renamed as HMS Rect-us.

All by assumption and presumption.

They never asked us.

Just 22 years later, in 1688, the Bill of Rights turns up and is now being used by common law fans to hold public servants to account.

That is, on account of the fact they have been wholesale raping us. To not put too finer point on it - as fines on us are the major game, of our id-entity theft.

By 1694 the Bank of England formed… and that, too, had us over when the private bankster families rocked and rolled up.

Suddenly we had spare cash for (both sides of the) wars - as has been the case ever since, if you care to look. There was not enough that we didn't board up the house... when the window tax came calling.

The modern version of this is 'council tax' - being as it is a fraud.

It has been systematically perpetrated by a private, for-profit, corp(s)oration, secretly passing itself off as:
HM Governments and Parliament PLC.

It's not just the councils that are 'avin a larf mate; they're all in on the constant cash in, and land grab and thievery - with their hand down the back of your sofa, your trousers and your kiddie's pram.

All of it based on 'statutes', not true law; while they hope that you don't notice that everything needs your consent - in plain eng-lish.

If it's written in 'dog Latin' it's not lawful. See Romley Stewart and his excellent tutorial to understand (and 'stand-under' jurisdictionally) what they really mean.

The biggee, of course, came in 1707 when the Acts of Union, kicked in.

Getting together with two great clans amalgamating.

We, the english, were then, free to travel unmolested and unlicenced cross border to Scotland to meet if we were lucky Nicola Sturgeon. If, however, Ms Sturgeon is not at home, but our luck is in, we could visit Clan McDonald standing proud in his kilt - with his ha' pounder on display.

Article 4 of the 1707 Act cannot be repealed; but that reality is regularly ignored by plod everywhere in Britain. Until we correct our standing and educate them on travel.

The next far from petty larceny occurred in the 1925 Lands Act, when that loyal, her maj. etc lot grabbed our property and landed us with the bill for maintenance.

We need to get back to allodial title, and look at what the sods have hidden from us. Soil and land title are most definitely not the same, my little fee simple-ton.

Now is the time to move from trust to allodium. That is full, not partial title based on:

1) full information;
2) intent;
3) exchange of true value;
4) fixed terms at the outset.

We think we have it bad in Britain but the Americans have had it worse; although they are fighting back, by reclaiming their political standing and with it their judicial power too.

On it goes year by year, state thievery, and criminality. It makes just as grim reading after the 'great' depression... as the grim reaper of poverty turns up in not so sunny 1933.

And in another bait and switch all Americans became bonded debt slaves. Their (creditor account) name, and (debtor account) surname pledged, as unwitting securities, for debt creation. Out of thin air, with only hot air to keep it floating.

Currency is printed but money is minted. Good as gold, we bought the ruse.

The UK wasn't far behind with the 1938 Bankers Act, and the administration bankruptcy of the UK.

In 1952 King George VI died and, as a respectable amount of

time had passed following the end of the spat between the German and British royal families, it was to be party time once more. The new monarch-to-be, was getting a new frock and her hair done.

Only bummer was… some jolly japers had stolen the stone. Of Destiny! Also known as god's witness, and if we lookey - no stoney, no crowney. All the invites had been sent out, though, with 33 Dundee cakes ordered. And 22 balloons.

What to do?

Sir Hector said, "I know, delay the corona thingy for 16 months so we can find it, and if we can't then ban the BBC from close-up filming. It's only a bit of rock - stone the bloody crows in the Tower, we're dealing with total in-breds".

The queen, likely, was in on the ruse stone - so on the 2nd June 1953 she autographed her oath, in purple (as us suverans do) but at the top of the page.

That way, above the text, she didn't 'stand under' her oath. Neat, yer maj. That private skooling wasn't wasted - clearly not.

She was at it again with her pledge to us; to serve "... in sincerity" or was it "... insincerity"? She should have said, to serve, 'in all sincerity', but likely she wanted her hands on our trust funds, so had to spell us and tell us.

Romley Stewart has spoken for countless hours on this stuff, the depths of deception, and he never bores me. He'll also let you know who owns Terra Australis... and it's not 'Australians'.

I'd vote him for King but, I'm sure, he'd tell us to stick it, down under.

By '69 it was all Lord Gardiner saying suck on this - as he repealed many common laws. Totally expected as a legaler, and we can add, unlawful, treasonous activity. He invented the wrongly titled 'law commission' under military orders. Sucking up to someone higher on the food chain - likely a traitor.

By 1971 many a curved ball was being bowled. From the grand lodge end no doubt. Bottoming out, as was his way, was spinmeister Ted Heath frolicking and staining on his Morning Cloud. The jammy dodger of deceit plumbed new depths with the EEC Treaty. A sold out, treasonous document, hidden from the people for 30 years.

Later that year common law was removed from the law society training/indoctrination. No wonder they don't know it - history re-written. Then, in ignorance, they arrest all of us: we the people.

Without 1984 where would we be, basking in vainglorious current covid-iocy? If the Control of Disease Act 1984 had been recalled we would be in a better place. Not up a gum tree without a paddle, as George Orwell had prophesised... this our must-have, inclusive, diverse and equal opportunity (for psychopathic leaders): covid-19-84 plandemic. Orwell got it spot on, in his '1984'. A bit more bow George - than boy George.

Meanwhile, in the mid 1990s up in Edinburgh Castle, a stone is returned back from the Sassenachs, albeit, since I tend to bitchiness (and accuracy) a much smaller one, and of a different colour, and not quarried from the same place, as the original. Is it?

Or so says Stephen Creilly and the original 1952 stone thief, Ian Hamilton. Now you're splitting hairs. It seems to be a shy stone too, suffering from acne - so no one is allowed to take a picture of it. The only object in the castle with such an order. Queenie, crowned, and not - in which order?

By 2001 it was cosy, cosy, tip-toe into more treason time.

There is barely enough to go round. The Treaty of Nice was now on offer. But this really was the final croissant that broke the camel's back.

Finally, the Magna Carta was dusted off, in english anger. Not all of it, but that most essential part - that of Article 61 and our Unalienable Right to Lawful Rebellion. (I prefer lawful dissent, but there you go.)

The invocation by the 25 Barons, enshrined for 800 years, was launched.

The queen returned her weak reply on the 39th day.

On the 40th day the invocation was served. She was stood down.

From 1971 to 2001 the cycle was complete; Treason against the people, it was.

It has got no better since, as in 2019/2020 the parliamentary philistines have claimed sovereignty. We don't even have a rudder, we have no ship, of state. Morally and mentally bankrupt, they have run us aground.

Pure and simple criminality and treason.

David Robinson is a name known to many in the constitutional and common law communities. Sadly, he passed away on 10th November 2020. Despite having been ill for a while he was still very giving of his time, and taught us willing neophytes a huge amount.

He also kept things simple.

Outlining the treasonous steps of Ted Heath in 1971, highlighted in the EU enslavement document: FCO 10/3048.

This dark arts secret was kept under wraps for 30 years, as the British people were sold down the river, and discussion denied by trendy luvvies and presstitutes.

This was compounded by the standing down of the Queen in March 2001 by the Barons, headed by Lord Craigmyle, under Magna Carta. Even the Daily Telegraph covered it. But along the way, the spine weakened of those trusted to speak out and to compel lawful action, as we slid more into the mire. Such is the way of life, but now, our time is here again.

David more than anyone, had extensively researched the English Constitution, the Magna Carta and the ensuing treasons along the way.

He was a kind and peaceful man, and resolute in his support for the Magna Carta's Article 61, that enshrining of 'Lawful Rebellion'.

David was kind enough to help me in the last few weeks of his life, to work on a document - which remains unfinished - as I stumble along.

We know his spirit lives on and like a wonderful phoenix, it continues to rise. We salute him.

In due course we will see rising, too, of New Nuremberg Trials.

With that in mind, the movement is underway towards true self-governance all over the world, as witnessed in Canada where the people are waking up to Justin Trudeau's malfeasance in public office.

Multi decade truth-teller and former pastor Kevin Annett is bringing to fruition the Republic of Kanata - via common law assemblies having previously highlighted intergenerational church and state genocide. Everywhere the crimes of the past are being exposed.

There are two kinds of people: those who want to be left alone and those who will not leave us alone.

Where do you think this next guy fits in?

Daniel Andrews is the premier of Victoria, Australia, who states,

"In fact, you'd be surprised at how much can be avoided, if people stopped insisting on their personal freedoms. Because insisting on human rights is not only selfish, it's stupid".

How do these guys get into power? It sure beats me. Given time, his robo-cops may beat you - for your own good.

If he ever comes across Tom Burnett or Romley Stewart on true Australian law, then I know who would win, if there was any justice. In plain sight and subject to independent scrutiny.

Their words are clear as crystal. That it's not only the dumb who use sign language - we, too, are all fingers and thumbs.

The Chicago manual of styles (17th Edition) makes deceptively easy reading. Deceptively being the key word and easy, only when Romley Stewart points something out.

Rumour has it, he took seven years to find this ultimate gem on page 666:

'one obvious limitation of the use of glosses from the spoken/written language to represent signs is that there is no one-to-one correspondence between the words or signs in any two languages.'

If we go back a page:

The sign for 'a car drive by' is written as 'VEHICLE-DRIVE-BY'.

In short, it's all DRVA (see 'Australia') registered commerce, so best stay fine free: as a traveller in your conveyance. In whichever seat you are sitting.

They say the eng-lish and the Americans are two nations separated by one language.

Much worse, legalese is a language that separates all and sundry, from their cheque (check...) book.

The good book, of course, makes no reference to the unalienable freedoms of:

1) cause no harm;
2) cause no loss;
3) keep the peace; and
4) act with honour.

We usually instead go downstream, where the waters and maritime courts are choppy and polluted.

The siren sounds attractive with her 12 maxims in law. These are all based on the person.

So, what is a 'person' then?

Funny you should ask; because it depends.

A 'person' is just an idea.

You're taking the P. When you look at your pass-port you'll see 'Type' P. I've been trying to unravel whether this 'P' means: peon, pleb, pawn or... person. But I'm recently told by a smart lady it means 'pieta' or pity in eng-lish.

To many, this word sorcery might seem rather anal.

But if it is person, let's look at how many 'person' definitions are listed in the latest, Black's Law Dictionary. In the 11th edition, on pages 1378 to 1382.

Here's just a few:

Person:	A human being - also termed natural person
Known person:	A person whose identity is familiar to others
Person not deceased:	Someone who is either living... or has not yet been born
Person of incidence:	The person against whom a right is enforceable
Private person:	Someone who does not hold public office
Protected person:	Someone who is protected by rule of international law
Artificial person:	An entity, such as a corporation, created by law and given certain legal rights
Fictitious person:	See artificial person
Public person:	A sovereign government
Personable:	Having the status of a legal person
Personality:	The legal status of one regarded by the law as a person
Persona miserabilis:	A pitiable person

... in short, me; after reading all this evil 'personal' deception.

The 2020 UK Coronavirus Act refers and applies to 'persons', and is not law. Just think about all the ramifications?

So, back to Maxims.

They have been handed down over time alongside common law. It would be in our own best interest if we ignore the countless legalers plying their trade using 'dead fiction' law books.

We can simply come back to (and I repeat) the four basic tenets of common law:

1) cause no harm;
2) cause no loss;
3) keep the peace; and
4) act with honour.

The following 12 maxims provide a picture of the tricks and tracks of life:

He who seeks equity must do equity.
He who comes into equity must come with clean hands.
Equity aids the vigilant, not those who slumber on their rights.
Equity follows the law.
Equity acts specifically.
Equity delights to do justice and not by halves.
Equity will not suffer a wrong to be without a remedy.
Equity regards substance rather than form.
Equity is equality.
Between equal equities the law will prevail.
Between equal equities the first in order of time shall prevail.
Equity abhors a forfeiture.

The following selection, though, may be more familiar to you:

No person shall be compelled to be a witness against himself.

We cheat, it is for them to find out.

Let all those who will be deceived, be deceived.

If you don't know your rights you have none.

The burden of proof lies upon he who affirms, not he who denies.

No man may sit in judgement in his own cause, or a cause to which he is a party.

He who makes the claim bears the burden of proof.

One who does not establish their rights has none.

However, these are all an inversion and perversion of the tenets of our unalienable freedoms.

The legalers have entrapped us by never making clear the fact that acts, statutes and codes do not apply to the living man or living woman without their free intent and consent.

And, let's be frank here, just because they make something illegal doesn't make it moral, tenable or defensible. At one time, remember, it was illegal to hide a Jew in your home.

This unlawful conversion is done via an unlawful trespass from the day you are born.

More so, when parliament tries it on, as 'that which we invented cannot be our master'.

In the key areas there is normally Latin, and the key phrase to note is: 'consensus facit legem' meaning, vitally, 'consent makes the law' which must - to be just - be fully informed and freely given by us. Consent makes the law - so, if there is:

no consent, no law; no victim, no crime.

It appears that there are two realms: the shadow and the substance; the rentier and the owned.

The realm of eng-land: of counties; and the realm of Rome: of post codes, councils, licences, and voting bind you into their lower realm.

So is it time to inform your local council / magistrates / merchants you have moved to eng-land and out of the sea? To require that they move you, out of their (claimed) jurisdiction.

Both realms may cover identical geographical area but they are different realms. Only one is eng-land.

The Editor in Chief of Black's Law Dictionary 11th Edition, published by Thomson Reuters, is Bryan A. Garner; so, let's see what he garners up... As we know that book is the legalers' guide to administrative hearings. So, the inside front cover has a pronunciation guide; ah... ah... or should that be aaargh, me hearties!

It comes with a disclaimer, warning that it was not prepared by attorneys licensed to practice law in a particular 'jurisdiction'.

Which is total b/s.

In reality, it's all horseshit and tram tickets.

It encourages you to seek 'legal' advice (in a 'law' book).

WTF? Front running the book, stock-brokers call that.

On page xiii Bryan confirms that he has been editing the Black's Law Dictionaries since the seventh edition, in 1999. Perhaps he daren't or won't recall about DWB (Driving While Black) which makes it into the 11th edition but not the seventh. Perhaps, one day, over vol-au-vents and champers, I'll ask him.

He didn't just lose me at hello; he left me all at sea.

Citizen-ship is, of course, that lost at sea status into which mums and dads are tricked into si(g)ning away their beautiful innocent offspring from the day when it is delivered on earth.

Shame on you Bryan, that you preside over all this criminal coercion and word-smithery magik on the masses.

Not content with being at sea some slither up on to land. A good number of these smug, supercilious, slippery buggers will get more than they bargained for in due course.

Maybe they should also read up on our not-so-friendly Mr Schwab's book, The Fourth Industrial Revolution.

In there he goes into detail about the cost-cutting and profit-boosting marvels of his brave new world.

He explains, 'Sooner than most anticipate, the work of professions as different as lawyers, financial analysts, doctors, journalists, accountants, insurance underwriters or librarians may be partly or completely automated...'.

So, perhaps the loss of jobs in the coming Great Reset is going to be affecting more than the plebs?

Learn to code legalers!

And remember, there are two kinds of people: those who want to be left alone and those who will not leave us alone.

It was at 11pm in March 2020 and I was closed for business. The door bell rings and it tolled for me, I had guests; but not invited ones. It was the boys in blue. Actually, to be precise boy and girl in black. There's one of each - a man, and a womb-man. Phew, my gender assignment coursework was almost complete.

The three of us started chatting, and as my phone video was working well, I captured the three-way interchange of the unfolding, and potentially entrapping, narrative.

Sadly, although the red light was a flashin', the ploddess - one Rebekkah Ringham (RR) it turned out - was not allowed by her handlers, upon later written request, to let me have her digital version. Due, it was claimed, to: digital/privacy rules. That's the: GDPR-B (General Data Protection Regulation)-(Bollox) rules to you and me. It seemed odd. Just me and plod plural. They should have been confidently two-up, as they'd started the match on their watch. Not mine - as I don't wear one.

Of course, particularly at that time of night, I didn't open the door. Although they were making sounds I did not clearly understand them.

Something about an issue?

I opened with, "Sorry, I'm closed for business, so what are you saying was going on?".

RR: "There was an incident reported earlier on today - we've just been asked to issue you with paperwork."

I requested they put the paperwork through my letterbox and said: "I am not conducting business with police or anyone who works for a corporation tonight. You're an officer, which makes you one of the 52 companies that operates on the Isle of Man.

The police service is a corporation, the prison is a corporation, 52 companies operate here, the schools are a corporation, it's in my book, From Health Heretic To Common Law Advocate.

May I give you a copy please, in the spirit of openness, that I gave to Howard Quayle's wife, round the back door? I gave them five copies, put on the floor; she's immune compromised, which is what my book contains."

RR: "I need you to sign it."

I said: "I'm not signing anything."

RR: "That's absolutely fine."

I then turned my attention to a man I know as Mark Hempsall (MH) and said, "We'll do a swap; we'll do a fair exchange, Mark. There you go, you've got two free books, I've got that [the document]. If you read it, you'll read, Who Is The Criminal? I make some fairly sweeping comments and accusations. There's something corrupt in the State of Denmark.

Matt Davison knows me. Andrew Lee knows me - he actually called me a c*nt in the police station... I was arrested four days before I actually tried to raise the HPV vaccine issues for boys; it is a crime.

Alex Allinson is a criminal, I have the evidence.

I have the clerk of tynwald folding my petition, that is a crime.

I loved the police in eng-land, I just wish they'd understand that they're working for a private corporation, and when they understand that we can all get on civilly.

I shouldn't have been arrested, I was 'driving' my Common Law Court listed conveyance, insured by Manx Cover, on 2nd July. I owned my car - you don't own yours, nor do you (pointing to RR). So, when you understand, when you regis-ter anything... you've given up your kids, you've given up your house, you've given up everything.

So if you want to go public, we'll put this on camera and that's the way it should be. Perfect, then we'll get jury trials not some bent bloody magistrate here or whatever".

MH: "Do you want to read those now?"

I replied: "No."

MH: "I've served them, they've been served. By the terms in there it says by a breach of them you could potentially be arrested. Have a read, it is self explanatory."

I countered: "This is the problem, that's what Hitler said before the Nuremberg Trials. People think they're going to get away with it. Every day you look at the sky - the lines across the sky are chemtrails, barium, aluminium, strontium".

I also stated: "I do not consider these papers served, I have taken them only in a spirit of openness".

Mark Hempsall also categorically stated: "I am only the messenger". His job being, at that time, Covid Team Leader and obviously just doing as he was told.

Amazing! Similar comments came home to roost seven months later.

In a Saturday morning email on 10/10/2020 I congratulated David Ashford, 'health' minister, on the award of his MBE. I wrote: 'You must be very proud'.

Within three minutes (literally) I had a reply:

'... I'm a bit shocked to be honest as I was only doing my job'.

Nuremberg Principle IV states:

'The fact that a person acted pursuant to order of his Government or of a superior does not relieve him from responsibility under international law, provided a moral choice was in fact possible to him.'

He has had enough emails, conversations and meetings to sink a Bismark of evidence. On my oath.

Further people 'just doing their job' had reared their ugly heads (and jackboots) back in July 2020.

This happened while I was working on a case with a mum whose estranged partner was trying to force multiple, catch-up vaccines on her young woman, called by some, 'A child'. The busybody location officers had even been round to con-fiscate both of their pass-ports two days before the online hearing. A hearing that was, at times, muted by the other side when mum made an interesting point in support of her daughter.

Their expert, one David Anthony Cyril Elliman, GMC registration 1643653, to me relies on baseless unsubstantiated and fraudulent vaccine science. I welcome one day facing him in any true court of record in front of our peers.

Unconnected with that case, on 6th July 2020 I was once more unlawfully arrested; that being my second consecutive tynwald day arrest. How darkly comedic!

In life there are spectators and there are participants, but you can't buy experience. Only many legalers and judges.

I had gotten it wrong letting my tendency for humour, ego and ignorance run ahead of me. Now I am only left with the letter plates, CLC JURBY.

My often ignored, and frequently wrong, wife is completely clear on why I no longer have the Renault Clio conveyance that was sandwiched between them.

Talking of being sandwiched...

I'm now at an age when reflection is in - even if the mirror needs a softer focus. So that we can face it. One such moment I reflect on, is our wedding day nearly 33 years ago. We'd been together eight years and it was time to make an (almost) honest woman of 'her', of my jude. There is, after all, only so much happiness one woman can bear.

We'd decided, or fate did, that 8th April 88 was to be 'our day' - a lump in the throat time. The location, as indeed fated, was to be the Isle of Skye. We were soon speeding on our bonnie boat, like a bird on the wing, over the sea.

On the way up we stayed in Glencoe - as stirring a place of cracks and crevices as you can imagine. Our senses were heightened as the sound of Billie Jo Spears blanketed the radio - me, her then Bonnie Prince and her, my wellbred easy spreading Flora. And to be up front, one day, if the postman had come just ten minutes earlier at least he would have had somewhere to park his bike. On the front lawn.

But, anyway, let's get back to my conveyance, CLC JURBY, for which I do have a one year no claims bonus insurance renewal certificate. From Manx Cover. In my name.

Since then I have reflected and replayed the scenario, of the role playing on the day. In my mind I realise my errors. In my dreams I now know the day could have unfolded very differently.

CLC JURBY revisited:

A policeman standing in the middle of the road directs me to stop.

I bring my conveyance to a halt and the policeman approaches me.

I remain seated in my conveyance.

The windows remain closed.

I turn off the engine and then activate the central locking.

The policeman attempts to engage me in conversation.

I remain silent.
(There is no requirement for me to answer any of his questions.)

He asks me to lower my window.

I do not follow orders. So I don't.
(I am not an employee of his corporation.)

He asks again, "Sir, you are not making this easy. Why don't you just lower the window it will help us?"

I again say and do nothing.

He persists, saying loudly, "We have checked the registration and there are issues with this car."

Again, I say and do nothing.

He persists, louder still, "Is this your vehicle, sir?"

I choose to lower the window a smidgeon, to help him hear me clearly say, "I do not answer questions."

His retort is, "Why are you being so obstructive, sir?".
(Using their neuro linguistic programming - NLP - training.)

Again, I say and do nothing.

He tries once more, "Are you the driver of this vehicle, sir?"

Yet again, I say and do nothing.
(As 'driver' and 'vehicle' are commercial 'for business' terms, and I was simply a traveller in my own conveyance.)

He says, "If you would just step out of the car, sir."

I reply, "Is that an order? I do not follow orders."

He says, "It's simply a request, sir. Why would you not comply?"

I ask, "Are you standing under your oath of office today?"

He says, "Sir, if you would please step out of the car."

I then ask, "Are you acting as a police officer or standing under your oath as a peace constable?"

He says, "Sir, why are you making this so unnecessarily difficult for yourself?"

I reply, "I do not answer questions. Are you now compelling me to answer questions, sir?"

He says, "No, but under the Road Traffic Act you need to."

I reply, "That is not a factual statement, sir. It is not correct."
(Any acts, statutes and codes can only ever be binding upon living men and women with their free, willing and fully informed consent. This is factual.)

He says, "Sir, can I see your driving licence to permit your driving of this vehicle?"

I remind him again, "I do not answer questions."
(I say no more than that, knowing he wants me to get in to 'controversy, argument and to undertake pleadings', any or all of which gives them legal joinder. Via unwitting entrapment.)

He says, "You just need to comply and stop being so awkward."

I then ask, "Has any crime been committed today, sir? Isn't it your duty to simply prevent crime and also to protect property?"
(That is all. Anything beyond is only for-profit, commercial over-reach.)

He says, "Sir, this is very frustrating and you're not helping yourself at all."

I reply, "Firstly, sir, on and for the record I do not answer questions. Secondly, I confirm I am most definitely not a 'driver' engaged in commerce and thirdly, for clarity, this is definitely not a 'vehicle'."

He says, "Sir, your belligerence won't change the outcome."

I ask him, "On and for the record, am I being detained to be later charged or am I now free to go peaceably on my way unmolested?"
(Simply based on the natural law tenet of 'no victim, no crime'. End of.)

He says, "Sir, you're being very combative... but there is no charge at present."

My final comment is, "Thank you for your clarity constable. I do not recall summoning you; you are therefore dismissed and free to go."

I turn the ignition key, start the engine and drive away.

There has been no contract, no joinder and no business undertaken that day on the Snaefell Mountain road.

It's a funny old game...

It reminds me, I'd once chanced upon a deemster when in a friend's court case. My friend was being progressed and processed through the system. Previously, fully in good faith, he had exchanged a half crown coin with a member of our legislative council, to seal a deal for where he lived. Deal done, or so he thought. Not so, apparently.

Some to and fro followed. Visitors came disrupting his peace, his non work haven, and outside of his sanctuary defined, convenient hours. Others, from their world of commerce, thought he was open all hours. He was up with the lark; they were up for a lark.

Some even forgot to note their meetings in their notebook.

Evidence is unsafe and unsound if not contemporaneously recorded and mysteriously omitted, m'lud. All or nothing seems a good adage for truth. Unless you've got a really good memory.

Before long, my pal and me were in court. We stood but others unsuitably commanded to sit, sat; and the clerk had grabbed his 'jurisdiction' by deception. Even an Oxford scholar was a-sat-sitting, on command.

When a 'hearing' is called a 'sitting' you should know it's because you really do... have no 'standing'. Last man to sit, and all that, in their lair, their legal realm.

Later, the local newspapers took an interest and wrote some words on common law, quoting deemster Needham who described it as: 'pseudo legal nonsense'. But in time, as is said, 'when the tide goes out we will see who is swimming naked'.

They, the journalists and the legalers may have some knowledge of common law, but choose to ignore it. As has the legaler profession which, since 1971, has chosen not to teach anything about common law.

If I may quote from page 13 of The Isle of Man Examiner of 25th August 2020. By Adrian Darbyshire:

'A Deemster has slammed the use of 'pseudo-legal' arguments used by civil litigants in the Island. Deemster John Needham took the unusual step of issuing a judgement to dissuade the use of such tactics which he said had no legal basis and were bound to fail. His judgement highlights the use by litigants of the UK based Common Law Court, which in an unrelated case last year saw health Minister David Ashford and public health director Dr Henrietta Ewart found guilty of 'crimes against the people'.

In that case, heard by the Common Law Court in Manchester Art Gallery last September, 'the people' were represented by anti-vaccine campaigner Courtenay Heading, a former Manx government healthcare adviser. He accused Mr Ashford, Dr Ewart as well as UK Health Secretary Matt Hancock and Jersey's Health Minister Richard Renouf of an abuse of position, criminal coercion and fraud by proceeding with the 'unlawful' use of the HPV vaccine.

The unanimous decision of the court was to find the defendants guilty in their absence of crimes against the people. It ordered them to be removed from their positions and barred from having any future roles in health. All HPV vaccines had to cease immediately until their safety was proven, the court ordered - and Mr Heading was to receive an immediate pay-out of £250,000, to be equally shared and paid by the defendants.

Deemster Needham's judgement came in a land dispute case where a defendant did not turn up for a directions hearing in the high court but instead sent a series of letters to the chief registrar in which she accused the authorities of 'entrapment' and attempted 'criminal coercion'.

The defendant who was referring to herself as standing solely under the jurisdiction of the Common Law Court, questioned the lawfulness of the hearing, asking: 'Are the Isle of Man Courts of Justice, also known as IsleofManGovernment, a private-for-profit corporation listed on Dun and Bradstreet? Is a legal fiction alive or dead? 'Are statutory courts unlawfully permitted to deal with living men and women?'. One of her letters had a Common Law Court Great Britain stamp at the top.

Deemster Needham said he was aware of the phenomenon of 'organised pseudo-legal commercial arguments' in which litigants put forward nonsensical concepts to try to claim that they are not subject to the courts' authority.

He said all such approaches, tactics, or arguments had no legal basis. And he warned: 'Pursuing irrelevant matters may result in penalties in costs, or even the imposition of further penalties for contempt of court if orders of this court are not followed. 'Ultimately, adopting such hopeless tactics may divert the litigant from pursuing any legitimate defence, which in this case, involving as it does the question of the Partition

Act, could mean the defendant losing her home. Deemster Needham said he raised these issues 'not to frighten or scare but to provide a 'sense' of realism' as to the important priorities for the defendant.'

~~~

(Please note. The above immediate payout of £250,000 was awarded to me on 1st September 2019 by the HPV vaccine harms jury. It was not requested by me but the jury's decision in recognition of my unpaid 'work' over several years.)

Pray tell, how far has all this controversy advanced us? Well, in truth, it has advanced a few at the expense of the many.

The shafter and the shaftee.

Especially now that Manx boys can get a dose of the vaccine for their cervix; coincidentally announced four days after my first arrest, in 2019, while wearing an 'HPV VACCINE DEATHS' yellow vest.

Alex Allinson (doing business as a GP, GMC reference no: 3483839) member of the house of keys (MHK) for Ramsey is currently also doing business as education minister. He is overseeing unlicensed medical experiments in Manx schools, one of which is Ramsey Grammar School. The current headteacher there is Annette Baker who, on several occasions, has declined a meeting with me to discuss this critical safety issue. However, any change in that role may find later, Sarah, that they are also criminally liable in their private capacity.

Under natural common law.

Some of you will remember Margaret Thatcher who, back in 1971, was the UK's edukayshun ministah when she withdrew 'free' school milk. All to save £4 million. From then on and for decades she was dobbed in and dubbed by the moniker, 'Thatcher the milk snatcher'. Hardly Hannibal Lecteresque, but there you go.

Nowadays, it seems to be okay to allow education ministers to inject bits of aborted baby, neuro-toxic metals, pesticides, insecticides and soon, agents that will make your kids glow in the dark. But no one looks at the recipe, preferring yet more blind faith. That someone must have all this covered. Dr Thalidomide? Perhaps, Thatch the Snatch wasn't so bad for the kids afterall. It's all relative I guess.

Who would have thought that less than 3 months later, by mid November 2020, Adrian's description of me as an 'anti-vaccine' campaigner would be tantamount to being called a terrorist?

Me. a terrorist? Come on, now. I mean, I may be many things but I'm no terrorist.

Well, that's what Britain's top counter-terrorism officer, the Metropolitan Police's Assistant Commissioner, Neil Basu, said. He has called for a nationwide debate on the introduction of new laws to punish people who spread anti-vaccination conspiracy theories.

He suggested there should be a discussion about whether it is, "the correct thing for society to allow" [people to spread] "misinformation that could cost people's lives".

He has clearly been given his orders, to add his two-penneth-worth to the mix, as there is a growing resistance by free-thinking and questioning people to this whole covid-con.

This swell of resistance by normal people, of all ages and from all levels of society, is likely to upset the protagonists' apple cart and will lead to undermining the voluntary take-up of any of the many (rushed and unsafe but immune from prosecution) covid-19 vaccines.

Now, I'm all for a debate; in fact, I have been calling for such a debate for many years so let's have one. Please. Recorded on camera by living men and women speaking in their private capacities under penalty of perjury.

Of course, there won't be.

It's just more blah, blah, blah by Neil Basu - repeating his masters' script - to smear those of us who don't buy their narrative.

When you hold a light to the darkness it becomes the one afraid.

So, bring out all your shaming labels: conspiracy theorist, anti-semite, terrorist - whatever.

Neil, you have been uncovered. We now know of you.

Maybe, in order to give a little balance, it might be appropriate to hear the words of a man who worked in a counter terrorism role in the UK:

'I am Ray Savage, a retired provincial UK cop. I joined East Sussex Constabulary (note the name 'Constabulary') as a Cadet in 1966. Constabulary as I understand the definition, was unlike Wikipedia today, a gathering of peace constables. East Sussex was a small, predominantly rural police area that served its inhabitants through a system that was locally accountable with a strong service ethos. This was portrayed in a commitment to the people. Crime rates were low, detection with community co-operation was high, violence was almost unheard of, murder a rarity, and the police public relations excellent.

When I started personal radios were not invented, and the oath I took was to protect life and property, and to prevent and detect crime. My motivation for joining the police was a deep seated feeling of wanting to help people, be of service, and to stand for truth and justice.

Whatever happened to this ethos when you see where we are today? I am appalled this morning looking at press reports of an incident in Bristol, where a 'reveller' was attacked by a police dog causing serious injuries that may prevent this individual, according to the report, from walking again.

I joined a service. What seems to have evolved over the interim 54 years, in certain places and at certain times, is a force whose ethos of service seems to have faded.

During my career, which was very varied, I did regular beat work as a uniformed bobbie, drove a panda car when the very successful Unit Beat Policing (UBP) system had been widely adopted. This system, provided a formula for the number of police officers that would be employed in any area per capita.

The police public relations, numbers of available police officers, and crime rates were some of the best that I remember. Apart from the cost it was never clear to me, why the system was disbanded.

A process of centralisation was under way at this time, under the guise of greater efficiency, cost savings and better service, whereas the opposite was true. Availability of money was primarily used, in the constant cuts in service. If one knows how money is 'made' you realise the nonsense of this argument. In my opinion this has been by design, even the change of name from Constabulary (Service) clearly tells us the change of direction that has been taken.

My career took me into the Training Branch, the Regional

Crime Squad, and Intelligence. On promotion to Detective Sergeant I ran a counter terrorist group at Gatwick Airport. I was also a uniformed section Sergeant in Crawley.

The training of men into riot squads started in the provinces in the late 70's. Prior to that, demonstrated well in the time of Mods and Rockers, the thin blue line, as we would have called it, was held by ordinary policemen without the need for the paramilitary look.

As a police instructor I was trained in Aikido, the martial art that held and dissipated aggression in its stance. This was the underlying ethos when confronted with violence. We were trained to contain and not perpetrate.

I ran a unit called the 'Heavy Mob' that was tasked with being a quick response unit to deal with any disturbances in Brighton in the early '70's. I would not have any violence perpetrated on anybody in the execution of duties of that unit.

Common Law was a subject that was taught on all initial training courses for police men and women when I started. We were taught the powers of arrest, and the judges rules that arose from Common Law. It seems that the police of today have little training in Common Law, as I was to sec later on the Isle of Man.

This fundamental lack of knowledge of the inalienable rights of all sentient beings.

I'd like to make some observations about our press. When I first started policing, the reports of incidents that took place in our locality were all logged in the station's Occurrence Book (well pre-computers).

The local press reporters would visit the station daily to ask what the news was. It was the job of the Station Sergeant or

Inspector to notate from the book what would be released to the press. Invariably this was taken directly from the Occurrence Book. There would be little censorship, only sufficient to protect individuals.

What I am saying here was a method by which the truth could be relayed and communicated to the public through the press. This process became centralised with a police Press Office at Headquarters and quite often, what came out of that Office was only a scant representation of the full truth.

Now we have media being used to perpetrate outright lies, and instill fear into the populace, which seems to be a way of controlling.

On the 6th August 2019 I attended a court case in Douglas, Isle of Man. I was present in the public gallery along with another former police constable who lives on the Isle of Man. We were there to observe the case against Courtenay regarding the travelling in his insured conveyance, a Renault Clio carrying the letter plate CLC JURBY.

After the court case, in the presence of the other former police constable, I chatted with the two police officers who gave evidence under oath that day. To me it was clear that neither of these younger police officers had ever been educated in Common Law. I sincerely hope this improves.'

~~~

Previously BBW (before book writing) I wrote a regular blog at jurbywellness.im on subjects as diverse as: the gut, mass screening, mental health, and the wise use of natural botanicals. The blog steadily morphed into an exposure of the major harms of statins, vaccines and anti-depressants.

With the disease-mongering-max of 2020 being pushed to

extreme levels of ridiculousness, my contempt for the medical business and 'health' industries has increased dramatically.

In most cases the unscreened live longer, while medicine ignores nutritional building blocks of health, habits and lifestyle. Sadly, but profitably. I think god must be bored with us.

I do realise, however, that I cannot fight too many battles at the same time. There are not enough hours in the day and most importantly, in truth, no one knows for certain how many hours or days one has left. This is true for everyone irrespective of age, gender, profession or status.

A friend regularly reminds me, "We're all going in the box".

This was brought home to me by a recent and what may seem flippant exchange.

I went walking with my walkerist friend on Sunday 15th November 2020, the day after I was per-mitted to leave my home following my 14 day covid-iot quarantine. It was raining and the wind was blowing a hooley while we did a brisk 13 miler. Around Maughold or, as incorrectly pronounced "Muff-Hold", by some off-island friends. Nope, one of them was not The Donald when forcing his attentions on the cool but rather cornered 'cat'... next door.

On our stroll we encountered a friend of mine leaving church (in muffhold). She, holding tight to her hooded coat in the rain, called out sarcastically, "It's a nice day to be out!". My walking friend, quick as lightning, pointed to the graveyard and proffered up, "Most of my family are buried there and they'd give anything to be walking in this". I added my nail into the coffin with, "I was on lockdown until yesterday". She got into her car and exited stage left.

My walking friend is right: life is fragile, uncertain and does not come with a money-back guarantee. If we truly understood this, we would be kinder to each other - and to ourselves.

It is unfortunate that, as is becoming clearer day by day to more and more people, there are some for whom kindness is the last thing on their mind. Their minds are simply too inverted and perverted.

Simply evil.

Their criminal activities result in untold harm, loss and destruction to the lives of literally billions of people across the world.

The reach and extent of the criminality is extensive. Once you wake up and get a glimpse of how things are really working and how you are being misled you can start to do something about it. Until you know, you can't.

Once you realise your own individual power, things can and will change - if you want. You will have to step out of your comfort zone, though, and go against the grain. It is not easy but as we've seen during 2020 our indivdual freedoms are being trampled upon, like never before.

It is time to truly make a stand. Not go on yet another march.

So Batman, what you're saying is, "It's like the withdrawal method, Cock Robin?"

Some religions practice the withdrawal method to stop pro-creation. Some folks, on the stroke, swear by it. Sweet Mother of Mary, maybe there is actually something in that? Actually, no, even if there isn't anything in the baby incubator, the fully empty womb with a view.

A shorter, simpler method is the wholsesale uptake of the HPV vaccine to induce societal infertility.

Is something or someone driving this agenda?

There are two types of people in this world: those who want to be left alone, and those who won't leave us alone.

As I've grown older, there seem to be ever more of the latter. Energy parasites, they are, too, but if we feed them with our attention, they grow ever stronger.

Ignore-ance is encouraged as their softskills weapon.

But, for too long, in my ignorance, I'd fought them, effed at them, moaned at them and ultimately paid a price in their, for-profit administrative courts.

Without success.

What they won't like is if we, in honour, leave their paper slave plantation. There comes a time, not just when silence is betrayal, but when we finally pack up our tent and go home.

Or, more accurately, we find our own way home.

It's a choice. Once you know and decide.

When something isn't right we can try and fix it from within. If it's so bent, buggered up and broken: start again.

So what does withdrawal mean? Well, it certainly means more than passive acquiescence of the status quo.

The key is to embrace non-violence; as violence is the state sponsored specialism everywhere.

John Lennon had it right, 'They know how to flick your beard to pull your hair, but they don't know how to deal with you, in peace'.

Most societies are struggling with state violence and infringements on our health, finances and freedoms. What if our roadmap has been all wrong? What if we have surrendered ourselves to the prison authorities, bought our own jumpsuit and paid for the guards and bars too?

I think the US spend of $16 trillion on 'covid' is slightly over the top.

I think most of us on the earth plane have been sold the wrong model; often, inadvertently, by our parents.

I think the Looney Tunes™ we've been dancing to have been well orchestrated but not in our best long-term interest.

Someone else is on the fiddle and conducting our dance band. While we bought the drinks and settled the bill.

All we seek is peace and harmony; well most of us, anyway.

Our life today is the culmination, a visible manifestation, of our previous thoughts.

Our ego tends to run the show. Certainly mine was, with a necessary Merc' on the drive and an Audi in the garage. Both, back then, quite vital tools for a happy and showy life.

Weekend washing and polishing burnt more of the candle of my life. Selling one bought me time, which then disappeared, while the proceeds were soon spent, too.

All too quickly I'd glossed over, 'that shrouds don't have pockets' as a friend said when he attended a funeral. If we're lucky we wake up before we hit the ground in a depreciation fireball.

That large mortgage is quite a fabulous tool for purchasing a well organised (but decaying) pile of stones. Who left that description out of the estate agents' briefing details?

Money is unreal and an illusion; it makes no sense, on reflection, to chase it up a blind alley. But we do. Money can't buy you more time, more health, nor more love. Although, as for love, maybe you will seem taller (and land that supermodel?) but only if you remain standing on your wallet.

So, how to start? How to cut loose and be a bit freer?

We're called human beings - but human doings would be more a lot more accurate. We don't like to sit still as it fires up the monkey mind, unless we've bet the well organised pile of stones (and the Merc') on 33 black in Vegas.

In the mind that's where we start, as everything physical flows from that. But it does come with drawbacks.

Ideally we'd all be rich in time, as on our death bed I doubt we'll be polishing our watch collection - as they empty our bag.

To have the choice of time and health is surely the greatest gift of all, especially when we're enjoying activities with our loved ones. That's what most of us really seek.

It's a bit of a game isn't it, aligning the mind?

Being the observer if we can - I'm certainly not able to advise. We only go where our attention directs us; but it needs constant vigilance. Often, the noisy chatter takes us far off course. Doesn't it just? It is from that chatter that we need most of all to withdraw. If we were to withdraw we might find true peace and harmony.

It's clear that our latest must-have enemy is something: unseen, unverified, without a post code, or a skin colour, or a sexuality, or political bent.

In short, an all inclusive wizard wheeze this: 'covid' caper. It's right on: inclusive, sustainable, diverse, one size fits all - it's a non-living 'virus' particle to scarily outsell and outfear all others.

It's spread and shed in over 200 countries by radio and TV - with knobs who set it to 33FM on their 24/7 fear-porn channel. But the viral load goes away when the batteries run down.

This non-visible, non-living 'virus' has, with a little help, shut down the whole world economy.

Just like Arnie, we've been told, 'I'll be back, but with a long Schhhwaaab'. To give us another wave or two, confining us to barracks, by force, in the place we used to call home.

Welcome to Our Brave New World, Mr Huxley.

If we withdraw, how will we benefit(s)? What will our friends say when we take a leaf out of Swampy's book and go live with him, up a tree?

Will it pain us when we take stock of all that useless, must-have stuff in the back of the cupboard? Might we feel the benefit of not just a spring clean? It could even oil our rusty hinges too. The electric salt and pepper grinders I saw on the telly on Come Dine With Me; well, they really took the biscuit. I never knew how we'd survived without them. Batteries not included, of course.

It all starts with the first step and the commitment, of course.

We'll remember first, to stand peacefully in our power - not bossily, but believably. We'll gain added strength by knowing no one, except the creator, ever stands above us. Anyone claiming otherwise is an imposter and an inserter.

We know true hierarchy because whoever claims the crown (or 'corona' in Spanish) on our behalf is handed a Bible - in Westminster anyway. Even if lizzie signed her oath (at the top) she knew where the true power lay.

Consent is all, and our withdrawal of it, is our first step - the reclaiming of our legal fiction name.

The second step is to undo the debt; the working-for-everyone-else-trap. That rampant feeling that if we own stuff, ever more stuff, then we're safe - but eventually it starts to own us and almost all of our productive hours.

When we sign up to vote we gift our 'power-of-attorney' to play by their rules, those of the state. They choose the pitch we play on as voters, often with a team sheet only they deem acceptable. It's time to manage our own team, Kenny, not just hand out the bitter lemons at half time.

You can try and avoid them all you like but sometimes the men in black do come calling. Late at night, when you might be closed for business. Staying calm and polite means they'll often be disappointed. They're only there for business - as we know.

If you don't engage and don't provoke, it's more likely they'll leave empty walleted. Rarely to return. Best of all, is to do your homework and respectfully ask them questions - but not to make claims, as he who makes the claims bears the burden of proof.

A big withdrawal is certainly healthy when it comes to medicine.

Don't poke the disease-mongering, asymptomatic screening monster and it won't poke you.

Fly your own plane and it'll serve you well. Especially if you maintain and fuel it well. By avoiding Dr Up-Seller his surgical skills may become blunted, or used on someone more gullible. Home is the first school. The first lessons learnt on the knee.

Malcolm X had it right, 'Why would you give your most precious gift to your sworn enemy?'. A bit strong but not a miss by a country mile. If you're looking for education don't expect schooling - which is quite different - to provide it. If educated a youngster can make a job, if schooled they can only take a job.

Might this lead to free-thinkers' anarchy? That would be a good thing in my opinion.

Anarchy.

Noun: "The absence of political violence, not the absence of rules. It is people organising themselves around principles without the use of force."

There will be anarchy, as defined above, when any government writes your name in lower case letters.

It's a work in progress to steadily withdraw from 'permission' permits and 'licentious' licences.

However, at polite dinner parties even raising such 'fanciful ideas' will see your friends wishing to unfriend you. Fine.

Who does rule over, and wish to 'reset', us then? "Mr UK that's who, Mr Pirbright." (refer to page 202 From Health Heretic To

Common Law Advocate.)

Taken direct from the Isle of Man government (gov.im) website: on 20/11/2020.

'Constitution

The Isle of Man is not, and never has been, part of the United Kingdom, nor is it part of the European Union. It is not represented at Westminster or in Brussels. The Island is a self-governing British Crown Dependency - as are Jersey and Guernsey in the Channel Islands - with its own parliament, government and laws. The UK government, on behalf of the Crown, is ultimately responsible for its international relations. The Queen, who is 'Lord of Mann', is the Manx Head of State and is represented on the Island by the Lieutenant Governor.'

Two simple observations in regard to the above:

How strange that the Manx police all bear .uk email addresses. Unless we are part of the UK, but are being kept in the dark by the men in black. Why so?

and

A bowel screening note plopped on my mat me being of a certain age; not so much for m'lud as m'anus. Again, it was received on island but was sent from a UK address. Why so?

For five years, I was healthcare innovation consultant to the Manx government. I had really hoped to do my bit. If Thatcher was not for turning then, I'd noticed that after five, up close and personal, years a government is not for changing.

At one 2015 meeting my government handler of the time was asked, "What will change?".

He replied, "Nothing; nothing will change".

He'd also told me around the same period (talking about the subject of the unnecessary deaths at Noble's hospital), "What went into the West Midlands Care Quality Review was but nothing compared with what was said behind closed doors".

A smidgeon in old money.

My later raising of that comment with him hasn't exactly brought us as close together as we once were.

If deep friendships come before truth then maybe we have a deeper problem. Even if we live, for certain, in the least bad place on earth. Along the way, if you know a Manx hairdresser or a taxi driver, you'll almost certainly know more than Dr Google. Or any dusty report.

All we have is truth, even in death.

And when it comes to it, this is the big one; which is how 'they' play their system, ply their trade and prey on us using our fear of death.

Fearful people are much easier to control.

Last year, out walking, we weren't even at Bride and the mad Manx monk was up and at it. It seems there are Four Noble Truths of Dhamma. The word dhamma refers to the truth taught by the Buddha. The image that springs to my mind (without knowing too much) is simply one of peace, tranquillity and reflection.

It is true that I know a lot about a lot of different things; however, if I am being truthful and reflective, my friend is patient with my ignorance about these spiritual teachings.

I do know, though, that the dhamma is learned through sustained practice. The practice of being aware of life moment to moment. This path or way of awakening is a gradual unfolding; it is a journey that is long.

The important thing to note is that no one else can walk it for us. A simple analogy is like walking the 85 miles Parish Walk around our beautiful island. We may have support along the route but you have to walk it yourself and bear your own pain along the way.

Each of us has a spirit, but it is so often buried - likely in a noisy, commercially-led world, and that's more than deliberate. But the spirit never goes away, it's simply behind our physical curtain. While we're distracted by girls or boys and toys.

As we age, hopefully we also sage. With luck.

Yet, as our body fades our softer spiritual being starts to come to the fore. As everything droops and stoops an awakening starts to happen; a gentle nudge that quickens. Well, it did for me, as the bell tolled around two decades ago.

Back then, the Merc' on the drive had lost its lustre. The physical stuff mattered less, no matter how much I polished it.

I was at an age when yoga was on the agenda, and event invites were on the mat, too. In short, physical and spiritual unity was, and is, where it's at.

But I had too much baggage aboard my plane, and it kept me in a low orbit. It still does, this circle of life. Is life.

What we start to do as we truly grow up, is try to create better experiences; ones that are invisible and light as air. On which we float. Private to us, but they touch everyone. Because what we do does touch everyone, even at a distance and they, equally, touch us.

We are looking for 'better' experiences. But better was not what I thought it was. Better was not external experiences, like wearing a posher suit - with the label on the outside. Who really wants to be a walking advertisement anyway?

Just what is that all about and how did we, me included, get so sold on it? We got told on it, repeatedly, then we got sold on it - that's how. Firstly, all softened up listening to compliance scripts, we were skooled not educated. That's how our soul decay set in.

I certainly didn't turn off the monkey, nor money, mind, allowing both to master me for a long time. The monkey still comes calling, but gradually he's being sent out into the cold, to stand in the corner without his nuts. But he's persistent and keeps banging on the window.

Only another trained monkey would put a noose around his neck, pay for the privilege, and not notice for 30 years. Oh, and by the way, anyone reading want to buy 100 of my old ties, made of the finest silk? "Suits you, sir; suits you." is now only on the nostalgia channels.

So, we all want better experiences, less angst and 'aggro' and, later, apologies. More priceless than a Picasso but saying it is the easy bit; detaching from the physical is hard. Someone needs to give us a proper internal - an in deep and personal 'internal inventory'. That someone is unavoidably us. No one else can do it for us.

Who hasn't heard that timeless saying, 'When the student is ready the teacher appears'. Spirit, in short, is what we pass off and call serendipity, not fully knowing nor appreciating that what we project, returns ten-fold. Or more.

I believe we are spirit having a bodily experience on earth. A decade ago, I'd known two friends for over 25 years but I'd never mentioned to them that I felt a deep-seated spiritual reality. Until, over Christmas, while sat in my own living room, I finally gave myself permission to do so. Mad isn't it? As in 'silly', the third meaning of that word.

They say there are three versions of each one of us:

1) who we think we are;
2) who others think we are; and
3) who we really are.

Simples, my little meerkat. Except it isn't.

It takes work as we labour on bumpy roads, around twists and turns - our life journey.

The ego constantly puts one over on us, protecting our shell like a crusty barnacle; the 'id' in our hard won: id-entity.

The Invitation was my ego wake-up call, and some.

Fast backwards 15 years ago and I was lying on a yoga mat in a monastery near Maidstone. Our yoga teacher was reading a soulful poem called, The Invitation, penned by Oriah Mountain Dreamer.

One line shot at me like an arrow:

'Are you prepared to disappoint another to be true to yourself?'.

Well, I've never been the same since. If I recall correctly, jude (my very own William Tell) got an eight page letter from me because of that one line.

183

"Yes...", was my answer, "I am".

Oriah reminds us to show up in the multiverse - to not flinch from, nor fluff, our sacred lines. Even if we stumble every day.

There are higher laws - natural laws - true principles, in reality, which transcend opinions and untested beliefs.

They help us move forward - if we obey them.

It's time we re-cognised the deep un-well we're in.

Then do something about it.

We need new myths and reverence to grow.

The hero's journey is to come home...

In that spirit, sorry seems to be the hardest word. If only someone bright had thought up those words - doubtless then they'd pen a hit song. Well, now it's my turn to say, truly, "I messed up, sorry, it's my fault".

Mea Culpa is an oh so handy Latin phrase for that working mens' shuv-ha'penny convention, in Skeggy. On reflection, it's increasingly clear that we are each just a fool; in short and in right royal parlance: jester prick.

Each of us has a unique song to sing.

As my walkerist friend says, there are 7 billion or so versions of reality; each one perceiving and experiencing their own unique world.

He also says, "You can't wake people up who are pretending to be asleep". Quite.

It is also said, 'The only thing constant is change'.

I originally thought that Father Christmas really did drop down my chimney and give me a hoop and stick and a piece of cheese, every 25th December. Until he didn't.

I also used to be believe that Lance Armstrong was a top bloke who suffered the pain of testicular cancer treatment, while having to contend with jealousy from the average cheese-eating-surrender-monkey Frenchman, as Lance peddled away in yellow. On steroids, blood products and, if legalers are reading, an untampered Mars bar.

He had his sorry session with Oprah. Mine was with Oriah. We all need to embrace a bit of sorry.

Sorry is one of those words apparently that crops up regularly on our death bed. Or 'death motorcycle' if I get to wish upon a star my ending, at: 120 miles per hour when 97 years old, in a spectacular pay-per-view fireball 'giving it large' on The Verandah.

Slightly more seriously, where to start?

Sorry may be cathartic but it is hard. It's simple but hard. It's ego limited and hard.

I've certainly known the cold chill of de-friending; most of it in the last few years. Caused by my mouth, which occasionally had been hard-wired to my brain, with a blown fuse, even when awake.

My wise owls say, 'It's a journey and you can't please all of the people all of the time'. Quite. But finding better ways so I don't pee them off so regularly would be a useful start.

The wise owls also say, 'Let go and let god'.

Listening more would be a great start and to remember we have two ears and one mouth. Fully guilty as charged - as reflections don't only appear in mirrors.

But most importantly, I've had friends who have, of late, whispered true kindness in my ears - plural - and, when that has failed, literally shouted at me. Deservedly. Especially, the long suffering jude.

My recent encounters with the police haven't helped. Sorry, as I do now think there is a better way; a gentler, more peeling back an onion education type way.

We're all just trying as best we can.

Thinking that others share the view we have, and prioritise it as we do, is a big mistake. One that is slowly dawning on me.

Sorry.

It depends on where we focus, which ill our ego choses to direct us towards. To anger us, and then feed that anger.

However, on reflection, as they say, 'There is no man so foolish that you can't learn something from him'. Or her, clearly.

If, as I believe, we each have a soul contract (a reason for incarnating) then, equally, we have a duty not to be rude and force-feed others with unasked for opinions. That was a truth gently delivered to me by a friend, most recently. Sorry, but I'd missed that.

Maybe I need to be more discerning as to who I vent at, but I cannot be so polite or sit back and say, "Of course, please do carry on with the napalming Bill".

Getting the balance right is the key.

Laying crumbs down to truth is a good start on ourselves - by stilling the monkey mind.

Was it really two decades ago that I glanced down at the pavement near St Pauls Cathedral. There was this inscription (but our friend Mr Google hasn't verified so I'm sorry if I get this wrong) to: Mary Ann Seeley 'Kindness dwelt upon her tongue'.

Clearly, painfully with me, that resonated. I need to learn to guard my tongue.

I also need to guard my assumptions and presumptions.

Last year, on 1st September 2019, I put the case for HPV vaccines harms to a common law court, when my standing was that of the plaintiff.

I was bringing the case against four individuals, and 12 good men and women true decided the case was proven; guilty as charged:

1) Matt Hancock;
2) David Ashford;
3) Henrietta Ewart; and
4) Richard Renouf.

However, plaintiff... is a legalese word and I didn't know that.

But it doesn't change the soundness of the evidence nor the facts of individual guilt - the slippery legalese words don't negate that.

The 'safety' trials for this toxic vaccine were fraudulent in every way and, as we know, fraud vitiates all that follows. Scrubs it out, in common parlance.

Since then, Matt Hancock and others have been at it again with covid-19-84. They, too, may utter mea culpa for their actions in New Nuremberg Trials.

Charging headlong towards the trenches, my eager-ness and my ego-ness made me do it.

Sorry.

As before, I had got my head up my anus - to be more than accurate. Speaking of which, just as I finished these words, postie dropped a note on my mat. Apparently, being of a certain age, I'm due my bi-annual inspection. I gather that bi-anal (in Latin?) means twice yearly inspection by the proctologist - so he can keep his hand in.

I'm sorry, mea culpa, very sorry - if I've got that wrong. Again.

And finally:

It's when we look back and wonder how we got here and how life passes in a heart-beat.

They say it is not the breaths you take but the things you did which took your breath away, during life.

One, for me, was seeing 160 mph on my Blackbird's clock on the Snaefell Mountain Mile in June 2018 - it takes some beating.

Heart beating.

Likely, in the two years since then, my cajones have shrunk, a tad, as I could only manage 150 mph in 2019. In 2020, of course, there was no chance. It was all covid-crimes-confidence tricksters; men with red flags walking in line to control our 'excesses', as anything above 40mph was deemed...

illegal.

All so the accident wards were kept clear, so they could keep the bullshit façade going of 'full' wards. Ones where a bored nurse plays TikTok and posts in-sync dancing videos to her just as bored NHS colleagues. At midnight. You've gotta laugh; god has been pulling my string in 2020.

In earlier years, there was also the odd trauma. Was it really 45 years since I took 'that' call? I knew as soon as the lady said where she was calling from - Thatcham - where my beloved, and still missed, Uncle John lived.

He had died suddenly, aged only 53. The first man who showed me how to live 'dangerously', when to tell lies about speed (but never to lie with malice) and how to light up a room when he arrived in a way that few ever manage. I can do that, too, but when I leave.

Also, he was the first ever deliverer of the immortal line, "She's as cold as a witches tit in winter!". To a pre-teenager, that had me rolling on the floor. It still does...

Form an orderly queue, please!

And most of all he was beloved by all who knew him. He worked from home, one of a rare breed in the 1960's. An artistic super-creative, whose architecture skills were only exceeded by his humour.

He packed a lot into those years, marrying a German lady. One smart move... after Zee Waar. Never did go with convention did John, and never ever a dull moment in his company. His sister, my mum, says I am more like John than I was my own father. I'll take a bit of that on a really good day.

As a sign-off for his life, too, I'm reminded of John's funeral when people laughed, but I struggled. I'm sure he sends me signals - the odd black cat walking across my path. I certainly feel his presence.

My dad, too, he showed me a sense of duty and sacrifice that few others would tolerate. He was from a more noble era - if a five hours per day commute, to help 'better' his family, could be called that.

Another major boyhood hero of mine was Jarno Saarinen, a name known mainly to motorcycle racing fans. Particularly older motorbike fans.

Jarno 'the flying Finn' was, at just 19, Finnish ice race champion. He rode a bike that, for near horizontal grip, had metal spiked tyres; the kind that if someone ran over you, you'd actually preferred they'd used a chain saw. For your bodily modifications there would have been less blood, and more to stitch together.

Proper hard.

Jarno soon graduated to road racing in Europe, and when that proved too easy, he plied his talents on the oval banking circuits of the US. On the way beating the very best despite others having twice the engine capacity. He upset the status quo and the apple cart in a massive way with his small bike... and less power... but far superior skill and talent. So, of course, and off course they banned him. Logically.

He was, and remains, one of the greatest riders of any generation. Living gloriously, he had made the same loan request story to four banks, but danced with them separately. Why should only bankers behave so 'creatively'. But he created without malice.

Kids throughout the world still carry his given name in

memory.

He died young, like so many heroes do, aged 27, due to the mistakes of others.

This is my 2nd and final book - of a four part trilogy.

I can guarantee some of you will have 'enjoyed' the journey with me so far and others will not have. I dare say those who haven't probably stopped reading a long while ago and aren't actually reading these words; however, we can be reminded of the last line from Theodore Roosevelt's poem, The Critic:

'... who at the worst, if he fails, at least fails while daring greatly, so that his place shall never be with those cold and timid souls who neither know victory nor defeat.'

I didn't have a plan to my life but others currently do.

They also have a plan for yours with covid-21 waiting in the wings, awaiting more cold air. Or is it hot air?

But, what if? What if a really good plan has already been done in Venus, Florida?

Jacque Fresco, was a social engineer. He died in 2017, aged 101, when he left the room in glory. Not a socialist, a capitalist, a fascist or a communist. He believed in people, seeing technology only as a tool; but not just for a privileged elite.

He didn't believe in restrictive college courses either; but in limitless expansion of individual potential. Working in harmony was his, oh so obvious, concept. He thought the great ills of the world were caused by social conditioning, by the schooling society in which we 'grow up'.

He lamented the 5,000 boats sitting at the bottom of the ocean, and 300,000 planes shot down. Caused by WWII. No, to be correct, caused by the utter ignorance of man: ill-educated outside of conditioning.

His Venus project in Florida lives on in testimony to the harnessing of technology for the good of all.

He had been shaped by the 'great depression' growing up in America. He felt that all governments were corrupt, simply desperate to cling on to power, using entrenched division and distraction and delusion.

People currently in the Manx government have trashed our economy, our social relationships, increased suicides, and murdered the elderly via medical ignorance. Others too.

The political cockroaches fear the torch of public debate - aided by the criminal cowards in the media.

For the young, the 'rulers' have destroyed all hope and nurtured the worst in our behaviour.

And still people sleep.

One friend has lost 95% of his travel business; he probably needs, as my walking friend observed, to lose the other 5% before he wakes up. Maybe.

No virus did that.

No mask did that.

Political reactions did that, aided by a sycophantic media and cowardice of the masses.

The m€dia is £he viru$.

The Manx Council of Ministers are bound by CR or 'collective responsibility'.

But four C's are better: 'criminal-cowardly-covid-collusion'.

They don't foresee the tribulations and trials that are coming. It has ever been so, while Herman the German thought the same in WWII.

The 'virus' is simply the cover-of-covid vehicle. This is the fourth industrial revolution, heralding in a new enslavement.

This is a perpetual, pre-meditated, assault on the spirit.

It is good versus evil.

Most of all, these sociopaths and psychopaths achieve their hidden aims because we are cowards.

People don't wear masks because they are afraid of a 'virus'.

They wear them because they are cowards.

Schooled in a restrictive vision of who they really are.

We are 'led' by visionless criminals.

The average MLC or MHK is that, at best. Average. Although their salaries do not reflect that fact.

Not one of them has a people-led vision. Not one holds anyone to true account. Mere posturing; more reports.

Rinse and repeat.

But now it's coming. We have new energy, new batteries, and new bulbs for our cockroach torches.

We must not claim our freedoms whilst on our knees.

We must live honourably.

We The People must: wake up, join up, and rise up...

In unity and peace we will hold a truth and reconcilliation event on Monday 5th July 2021.

Please come.

courtenay-adam-lawrence

Isle of Man
20/11/2020

PS.

'coronavirus' =

your own amplified DNA...

your very own: Ch£omo$om€ 8

(Defined in the WHO homo sapiens, test primer protocol, sequence: CTCCCTTTGTTGTGTTGT)

You can contact me via:

courtenay@manx.net

or

courtenay@jurbywellness.im

website:
www.jurbywellness.im

The Con.

No Virus;

No Test;

No Contagion.

"That's all Folks!"

In deference to:
Looney Tunes™